NCCN Guidelines for Patients®

The essential guide for people facing cancer.

Based on care recommendations from leading cancer experts.

Explains high-quality cancer care provided at state-of-the-art cancer centers.

Reviewed and revised every year.

Did you know that top cancer centers across the United States work together to improve cancer care? This alliance of leading cancer centers is called the National Comprehensive Cancer Network® (NCCN®).

Because cancer care is always evolving, NCCN develops and frequently updates evidence-based cancer care recommendations used by health care providers worldwide. These recommendations are known as the NCCN Clinical Practice Guidelines in Oncology (NCCN Guidelines®).

The NCCN Guidelines for Patients plainly explain these expert recommendations, so you can talk with your care team about the best care for you.

These NCCN Guidelines for Patients are based on the NCCN Guidelines® for Pediatric Acute Lymphoblastic Leukemia Version 1.2026 – August 11, 2025.

View the NCCN Guidelines for Patients free online: NCCN.org/patientguidelines

Find an NCCN Cancer Center near you: NCCN.org/cancercenters

Learn how the NCCN Guidelines for Patients are developed: NCCN.org/patient-guidelines-process

Connect with us

@NCCNorg @NCCNVideo NCCN @NCCNorg

Supporters

NATIONAL COMPREHENSIVE CANCER NETWORK®
NCCN FOUNDATION
Guiding Treatment. Changing Lives.

NCCN Guidelines for Patients are supported by funding from the NCCN Foundation®

NCCN Foundation gratefully acknowledges the following corporate supporters for helping to make available these NCCN Guidelines for Patients: Amgen Inc.

NCCN independently adapts, updates, and hosts the NCCN Guidelines for Patients. Our corporate supporters do not participate in the development of the NCCN Guidelines for Patients and are not responsible for the content and recommendations contained therein.

To make a gift, visit
NCCNFoundation.org/Donate

To learn more, visit online
NCCN.org/patientguidelines
or email
PatientGuidelines@NCCN.org

Contents

NCCN Foundation seeks to support the millions of patients and their families affected by a cancer diagnosis by funding and distributing NCCN Guidelines for Patients. NCCN Foundation is also committed to advancing cancer treatment by funding the nation's promising doctors at the center of innovation in cancer research. For more details and the full library of patient and caregiver resources, visit NCCN.org/patients.

National Comprehensive Cancer Network (NCCN) and NCCN Foundation
3025 Chemical Road, Suite 100, Plymouth Meeting, PA 19462 USA

1

About ALL

Acute lymphoblastic leukemia (ALL) is the most common cancer that children get. It's a cancer that starts in lymphocytes (a type of white blood cell that develops in the bone marrow). What treatment your child receives depends on the type of ALL they have, their age at diagnosis, and other factors. This guide covers treatment for ALL in infants, children, and young adults.

What's in this guide?

This guide describes everything you need to know about pediatric ALL, including:

- Tests needed to figure out the best treatment for your child
- The different phases of treatment (there are usually 3: induction therapy, consolidation therapy, and maintenance therapy)
- Treatments available for the different subtypes of ALL
- Supportive care to improve your child's quality of life

What is ALL?

Acute lymphoblastic leukemia (ALL) is a blood cancer that starts in disease-fighting white blood cells called lymphocytes. Lymphocytes are part of our immune systems. They help our bodies fight infections. Like other blood cells, lymphocytes are made in our bone marrow (the spongy tissue in the center of most bones).

However, in people with ALL, the bone marrow makes too many immature lymphocytes called lymphoblasts (or blasts). Lymphoblasts can't fight infections, and because they crowd out other blood cells, the bone marrow isn't able to work right.

There are 2 main types of ALL:

- B-cell (B-ALL)
  - Affects B lymphocytes (B cells), which make antibodies. An antibody protects us when unwanted substances enter our bodies.
- T-cell (T-ALL)
  - Affects T lymphocytes (T cells), which help fight infections and kill tumor cells.

What is pediatric ALL?

Pediatric ALL is ALL that occurs in infants, children, and young adults. This includes anyone who's 18 years of age or under, and certain adolescents and young adults (AYAs) over 18 years of age. People who are AYAs are 15 to 39 years of age when they're diagnosed with cancer. They can receive treatment in a pediatric or adult cancer center depending on what type of cancer they have. This guide is for children and AYAs who are being treated at a pediatric or children's cancer center who are 30 years of age or under.

Information for people being treated for ALL at an adult cancer center can be found in *NCCN Guidelines for Patients: Acute Lymphoblastic Leukemia* available at NCCN.org/patientguidelines and on the NCCN Patient Guides for Cancer app.

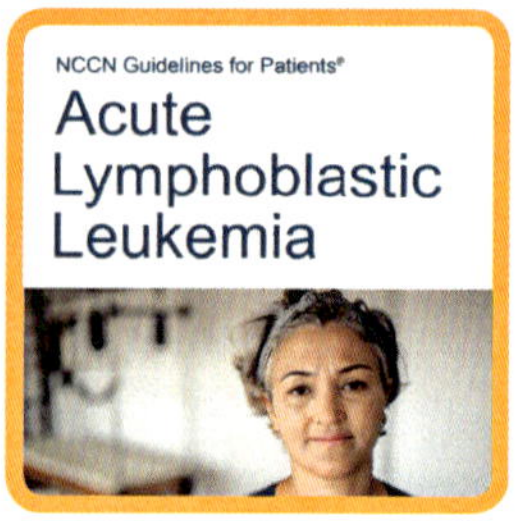

What is the B-ALL subtype of ALL?

B-ALL is the most common type of pediatric ALL. It starts in immature B-cell lymphocytes. Treatments for B-ALL depend on whether leukemia cells have the *BCR::ABL1* gene, also known as the Philadelphia chromosome, so it's important for your child's care team to figure out exactly what type of B-ALL they have.

There are 2 main types of B-ALL:

- *BCR::ABL1*-positive B-ALL
- *BCR::ABL1*-negative or *BCR::ABL1*-like B-ALL

Children with *BCR::ABL1*-positive B-ALL have leukemia cells with the *BCR::ABL1* gene and children with *BCR::ABL1*-negative B-ALL don't have the gene in their leukemia cells. The *BCR::ABL1* gene is an abnormal gene in leukemia cells that's formed when parts of the BCR gene and *ABL1* gene join together to make something called a fusion gene. *BCR::ABL1*-like B-ALL is when the cancer cells look like the *BCR::ABL1* gene is there even though it isn't.

Types of ALL

- B-ALL
  - *BCR::ABL1*-positive B-ALL
  - *BCR::ABL1*-negative or *BCR::ABL1*-like B-ALL
- T-ALL
- Infant ALL

Importantly, treatments for *BCR::ABL1*-positive B-ALL are not always the same as treatments for *BCR::ABL1*-negative and *BCR::ABL1*-like B-ALL. *Chapter 6: Treatments for* BCR::ABL1-*negative or* BCR::ABL1-*like B-ALL* describes the treatments your child will get if they have *BCR::ABL1*-negative or *BCR::ABL1*-like B-ALL. *Chapter 7: Treatments for* BCR::ABL1-*positive B-ALL* describes the treatments for the *BCR::ABL1*-positive type of B-ALL.

What is the T-ALL subtype of ALL?

T-ALL starts in immature T-cell lymphocytes. Because T-ALL and B-ALL are different types of ALL, a treatment that works for someone with B-ALL might not work the same way for someone with T-ALL. So, treatments for T-ALL can be different from treatments for B-ALL. *Chapter 8: Treatments for T-ALL* describes what treatments your child will get if they have this subtype.

What is infant ALL?

Infant ALL is when children under 1 year old have ALL. Treatment for infant ALL is different from treatment for children who are 1 year old and older. Infants receive therapy based on if a gene called *KMT2A* is rearranged. The options are explained in *Chapter 9: Treatments for infant ALL*.

How is pediatric ALL identified?

Pediatric ALL is often found when certain **symptoms** occur. A symptom is a feeling someone has that can be a sign of a disease or condition. Symptoms of pediatric ALL can include feeling tired (fatigue), fevers, night sweats, weight loss, shortness of breath, dizziness, infections, looking pale, and bruising or bleeding easily.

Children might only feel painful symptoms in their joints or arms and legs. Additionally, if the nervous system is involved, numbness in the chin or weakness in the muscles on 1 side of the face can also be signs of ALL. Testing will confirm if your child has ALL (tests are described in *Chapter 2: Testing for ALL* and *Chapter 3: Testing to plan treatment*).

How is pediatric ALL treated?

All children with ALL are treated with a combination of various chemotherapies. The specific chemotherapy drugs and treatments your child gets will be the ones that work best for their type of ALL. Importantly, all treatment plans include a type of chemotherapy called intrathecal chemotherapy. This type of chemotherapy is injected into your child's spinal fluid, so it can reach the brain and spinal cord. It's given to prevent and treat cancer in the nervous system and brain.

Other treatments your child might get are targeted therapy (a type of treatment that targets specific or unique features of cancer cells), a hematopoietic cell transplant (also known as a stem cell or bone marrow transplant), and treatment in a clinical trial (a type of medical research study that looks at new ways to fight cancer).

Your child will receive treatment in different phases, which are described in *Chapter 5: Phases of treatment*. There 3 main phases of treatment are induction therapy, consolidation therapy, and maintenance therapy.

Your child's care team

Treating ALL takes a team approach. Your child's care team will include different health care professionals who are experts in pediatric ALL. Some members of your child's care team will be with you throughout cancer treatment, while others will only be there for parts of it. Get to know your child's care team and help them get to know you and your child.

Supportive care: Help during and after treatment

Supportive care is an important part of cancer care. It includes many different services, such as palliative care. The goal of supportive care is to improve your child's quality of life during and after cancer treatment. *Chapter 10:*

Supportive care describes more about what supportive care is and how it can help.

How can my child get the best care?

Advocate for yourself and your child. You have an important role to play in your child's care. Many people feel more satisfied when they actively take part in planning their child's cancer care.

The NCCN Guidelines for Patients will help you play a larger role in care. Discuss the recommendations in this guide with your child's care team. Ask questions about options and share your goals and concerns.

Don't know what to ask? You're not alone. That's why we include suggested questions to ask at the end of chapters.

Keep reading to find the best care for your child.

How this guide can help you

Making decisions about cancer care is stressful. There's a lot to learn, and you don't know what the future holds.

Use this guide to get the information and support you need.

Patients, doctors, and other health care professionals trust the NCCN Guidelines for Patients. This guide uses clear, everyday language to explain current cancer care recommendations made by respected experts in the field. Their recommendations are based on the latest research and practices at leading cancer centers.

Your child's health is unique, so their cancer care should be, too. As you read this guide, you'll learn which treatments are likely to provide the best results. And you'll be better prepared to talk with your child's care team.

2

Testing for ALL

Accurate testing is needed to diagnose (confirm) and treat acute lymphoblastic leukemia (ALL). This chapter explains the tests used to diagnose ALL and what to expect.

In general, to diagnose someone with acute lymphoblastic leukemia (ALL), at least 1 out of 5 of their bone marrow cells must be lymphoblasts.

The tests used to diagnose ALL can be found in **Guide 1**.

Bone marrow tests

Leukemia starts in the bone marrow, which is the spongy tissue in the center of most bones where blood cells (like lymphocytes) are made. To diagnose ALL, samples of bone marrow must be removed and tested. Although this can sometimes be a painful procedure, your child's care team will try to make them as comfortable as possible. Some health centers will give your child a sedative drug (makes someone calm and drowsy) or anesthesia (puts someone to sleep) for this procedure.

Guide 1 **Tests and procedures done to diagnose pediatric ALL**
Bone marrow aspiration and biopsy
Immunophenotyping test

There are 2 types of bone marrow tests that are often done at the same time:

- Bone marrow aspiration
- Bone marrow biopsy

A bone marrow biopsy removes a sample of solid bone marrow. A bone marrow aspiration removes liquid bone marrow. Both bone marrow samples are usually taken from the back or front of the hip bone at the same time. Importantly, not everyone with ALL will get a bone marrow biopsy, but everyone will get a bone marrow aspiration.

After the samples are taken, they'll be sent to a lab for testing. The bone marrow sample will be reviewed by a hematopathologist who is an expert in diagnosing ALL.

Immunophenotyping test

Immunophenotyping is a very important test that tells your child's care team if they have ALL or a different type of leukemia. Your child's care team will do detailed (comprehensive) immunophenotyping, which will show if your child has B-cell or T-cell ALL. Immunophenotyping examines something called a leukemic clone, which is a group of identical cancer blood cells that all come from the same mutated cell.

The test finds certain proteins called antigens on white blood cells. These antigens can be **biomarkers** (also called biological markers or markers). Biomarkers are used to figure out what treatment may work best for your child. Some treatments today target specific biomarkers to treat people with cancer who have that particular biomarker.

Your child's care team will look at the cancer cells when your child is diagnosed with ALL, so the findings can be used as a baseline for later. After some treatment, their care team will look to see if the number of cancer cells has decreased.

Testing for ALL biomarkers and genetic changes

Genetic tests are used to learn more about your child's type of ALL. Your child's leukemia cells will be tested for genetic changes that are not in the other cells in their body. After genetic testing is done on your child's bone marrow, the test results will help their care team place them into a risk group. Treatment for ALL is given based on if they have standard-risk or high-risk ALL and is also based on what type of ALL they have.

ALL mutation testing

The methods your child's care team will use to look for genetic changes (abnormalities) in the leukemia cells include karyotyping of specific chromosomes, interphase fluorescence in situ hybridization (FISH) testing, reverse polymerase chain reaction (PCR) testing, and next-generation sequencing (NGS) testing.

A sample of your child's blood, bone marrow, or in some cases a swab of their mouth or nose will be used for the tests. More tests or assessments may be done in some cases, and a whole transcriptome sequencing test might be needed to find certain subtypes of ALL.

Bone marrow biopsy

Doctors use a bone marrow biopsy and aspiration to remove samples of solid bone marrow and liquid bone marrow for testing. These tests are often done at the same time on the pelvic bone.

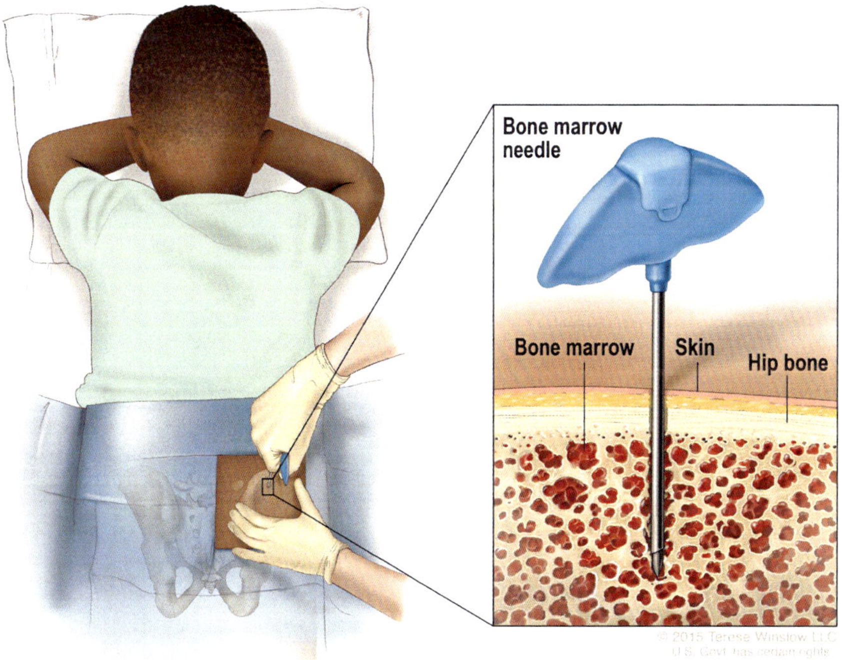

What are DNA and chromosomes?

DNA molecules are inside of our cells and are tightly packaged into what is called a chromosome. Chromosomes contain most of the genetic information in a cell, and each chromosome contains a lot of genes. Genes give our bodies instructions to make proteins. Proteins make our bodies work the right way. A mutation is a change or mistake in a gene's DNA.

Karyotyping

A karyotype is a picture of all of someone's chromosomes. Normal human cells have 23 pairs of chromosomes, for a total of 46 chromosomes. Leukemia cells can have changes to the normal number or order of chromosomes. A karyotype will show any extra, missing, rearranged, or abnormal pieces of chromosomes in your child's leukemia cells. To make a karyotype, your child's care team will take a blood or body fluid sample from them.

FISH testing

FISH testing can find gene changes that are amplifications, translocations, rearrangements, and deletions. However, it cannot detect all of the possible changes found within genes or chromosomes.

NGS testing

NGS testing is used to figure out the sequence (order) of someone's DNA. It can find mutations and changes in genes. NGS looks at the genes in a more detailed way than other testing methods and can find mutations that other methods might miss.

PCR testing

A PCR test creates more copies of DNA so that the DNA can be better examined. It can find genetic changes and help diagnose ALL.

Key points

- ALL is diagnosed (confirmed) using a bone marrow aspiration with or without a bone marrow biopsy. Other tests can also be done to help with the diagnosis.
- Immunophenotyping is a very important test that tells your child's care team if they have ALL or a different type of leukemia.
- Genetic and biomarker tests are done to learn more about your child's ALL and to figure out what subtype of ALL they have. These tests will likely guide the care team when picking treatments.

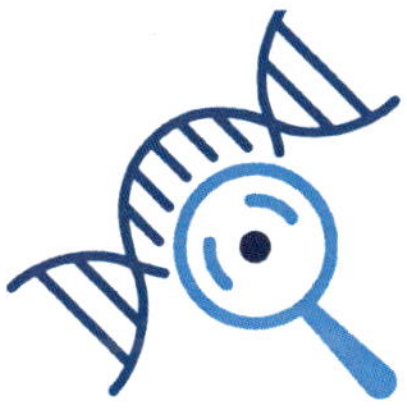

ALL genetic changes

Many people with ALL have genetic changes in their leukemia cells. A genetic change is when the order of DNA in your genes changes. Genes are pieces of DNA that give your cells instructions for certain traits or body functions.

Some genetic changes make cancer respond better to treatment than other genetic changes. Additionally, certain treatments target specific genetic changes. Therefore, it's important to know if your child has any genetic changes and if they do, what the changes are. Here are some types of genetic changes that can happen:

- **Amplification** – When there is an increase in the number of copies of a gene.
- **Deletion** – When a section of DNA is lost or deleted.
- **Insertion** – When a new piece of DNA is added.
- **Translocation** – When a chromosome (strings of DNA wrapped around proteins) breaks, and the broken-off pieces reattach to other chromosomes.
- **Rearrangement** – When there is a change in the structure of a chromosome. Pieces of the chromosome could be moved around, missing, or there could be extra pieces.

Questions to ask

- Who will explain my child's test results to me and when?
- Will my insurance pay for these tests?
- What happens after my child is diagnosed with ALL?
- What other tests will my child need and when will they get them?
- Is there a cancer center or hospital nearby that specializes in this cancer?

What's next?

After your child is diagnosed with pediatric ALL, their care team will do some more tests to learn more about the ALL and how to treat it. The additional tests your child might receive are explained in the next chapter.

3

Testing to plan treatment

After your child is diagnosed with ALL, they'll need to have a few more tests done. These tests will help their care team learn more about their ALL and how to best treat it.

The tests and procedures your child will get after receiving a pediatric ALL diagnosis are listed in **Guide 2**. Additional tests that might be done are explained later in the chapter and in **Guide 3**. The results from blood tests, bone marrow tests, and imaging scans will be used to help determine your child's treatment plan.

Guide 2 **Tests and procedures done to plan and prepare for pediatric ALL treatment**
Medical history and physical exam
Complete blood count, differential, chemistry profile, and liver function tests
Tumor lysis syndrome panel examining levels of lactate dehydrogenase, uric acid, potassium, calcium, and phosphorus
Chest x-ray to rule out a mass between the lungs (mediastinal mass)
Lumbar puncture (spinal tap) with intrathecal chemotherapy
Central venous access device of your choice (allows your child's care team to give them fluids, blood products, medication, and more)
Assessment for predisposition syndromes (genetic conditions that can increase someone's risk of developing a disease such as cancer) which include: • Down syndrome (also called trisomy 21) • *TP53* variants for certain children (children with a low number of chromosomes) • The *PAX5*, *ETV6*, and *IKZF1* variants, which are associated with developing B-ALL • Having another cancer (ALL can be a second cancer)
Pharmacogenomic testing to look for certain genetic changes (the *TPMT* and *NUDT15* variants)
Bleeding and clotting examination which includes: • A DIC panel that looks at D-dimer level, fibrinogen level, prothrombin time (blood clotting time), and partial thromboplastin time (blood clotting time)
A psychosocial assessment is encouraged to figure out how your child is doing mentally, emotionally, and socially

Medical history

Your child's care team needs to have all of their health information. They'll ask you about any symptoms, health problems, and treatments your child has had. A complete report of their health is called a medical history.

When you meet with the care team, be ready to talk about your child's:

- Illnesses
- Surgeries
- Injuries
- Health conditions
- Symptoms
- Medications and supplements

Family history

Your child's care team will also ask about the health history of family members who are blood relatives. This information is called a family history. If any family member has had cancer, it's important to know the specific type of cancer, where the cancer started, and if it's in multiple locations. It's also important to find out if they had genetic testing done.

A complete family history can help tell if your child could have a cancer predisposition syndrome. A cancer predisposition syndrome is a genetic mutation that someone inherits that can increase their risk of developing cancer.

"If your child's care team starts explaining things that are hard to understand, don't hesitate in asking questions. Ask them to slow down and re-explain, and don't feel bad about it."

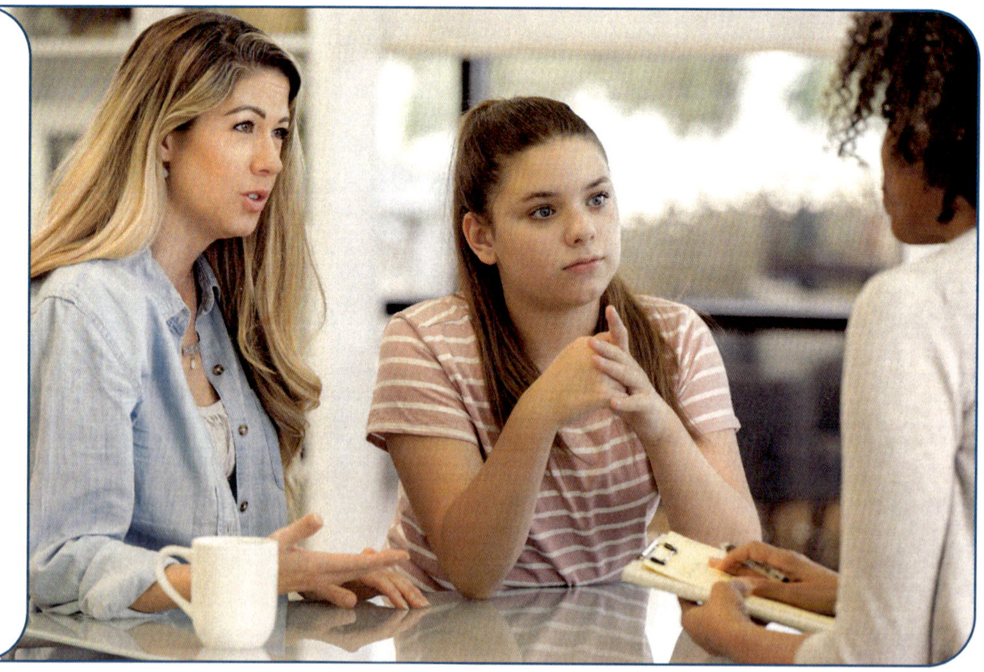

Physical exam

A physical exam is done to look for signs of cancer. During this exam, your child's doctor or health care professional may check their:

- Temperature, blood pressure, pulse, oxygen saturation, and breathing rate
- Height and weight

They will also:

- Listen to their lungs, heart, and gut
- Look at their eyes, skin, ears, nose, and mouth
- Feel and apply pressure to parts of their body to see if organs are a normal size or if there's pain when touched
- Do a testicular exam if they were born with male sex organs
  - A testicular exam may be done in certain cases because B-ALL can sometimes involve the testicles. A scrotal ultrasound might also be done.

Blood tests

Blood tests check for signs of disease and can help show how well organs are working. A blood draw is done by inserting a needle into a vein to remove some of your child's blood for testing.

These are the tests that may be done with the blood sample:

Complete blood count with differential

A complete blood count measures parts of the blood, including white blood cells, red blood cells, and platelets. A differential counts the number of each type of white blood cell. A differential can also show if there are too many immature white blood cells (lymphoblasts or blasts) in the blood. Cancer and other health problems can cause low or high counts. This test will be done before, during, and after treatment to check on your child's blood counts.

Chemistry profile

A chemistry profile or panel measures the levels of different substances in your child's body. These substances include proteins, enzymes, and sugars. If your child has ALL, the chemistry panel might look different from the way it normally would.

Liver function tests

Liver function tests look at the health of the liver by measuring substances that are made or processed by the liver. Too much or not enough of certain substances can be signs of an illness, injury, or disease.

Tumor lysis syndrome panel

Cancer treatment kills cancer cells in the body and sometimes causes tumor lysis syndrome as a result. Tumor lysis syndrome occurs when the substances released by the dead cells build up faster than the body can get rid of them.

Changes in potassium, phosphorus, calcium, creatine, and uric acid levels can be signs of tumor lysis syndrome. A tumor lysis syndrome panel examines these levels and levels of other substances, such as lactate dehydrogenase. Levels are watched closely when your child is first diagnosed with ALL. Your child can also receive medicine and intravenous (IV) fluids to help prevent the levels from getting too high.

Blood clotting tests

Your body stops bleeding by turning blood into a gel-like form. The gel-like blood forms into a solid mass of blood called a blood clot. In very uncommon cases, leukemia can affect the blood clotting process and can cause a disorder called disseminated intravascular coagulation, which results in uncontrolled clotting.

To test for this, a disseminated intravascular coagulation (DIC) panel may be done. This is a test that examines several things that impact blood clotting, including D-dimer level, fibrinogen level, and blood clotting time (prothrombin time and partial thromboplastin time).

Lumbar puncture with intrathecal chemotherapy

Leukemia can travel to the fluid that surrounds the spine and brain (cerebrospinal fluid). A lumbar puncture (also called a spinal tap) is done to see if the cancer has spread to those areas.

A lumbar puncture is a procedure that removes spinal fluid. To look for leukemia cells in your child's brain and spinal fluid, a sample of the fluid must be taken and then tested. A lumbar puncture is also used to inject chemotherapy into spinal fluid and is required throughout ALL therapy. This is called intrathecal chemotherapy. All treatment plans for ALL include intrathecal chemotherapy, even if no leukemia cells are found in the spinal fluid.

Central venous access device

Your child will receive a central venous access device, which allows their care team to give them fluids, blood products, medication, and more. The device is a catheter (thin tube) that is inserted into a vein. Different devices include port-a-caths (ports) or peripherally inserted central catheter (PICC) lines, among other types. When your child's care team needs to test their blood, they can also do a blood draw (take a sample of their blood) using the central venous access device.

Pharmacogenomic testing

Pharmacogenomics is the study of how a person's genetic makeup affects their response to medicines and drugs. How well your child's body absorbs and processes medicine is an important factor in treatment.

Therefore, your child's care team may do a genetic test on your child's regular (not leukemia) cells to find the best starting dose of certain drugs. For ALL, pharmacogenomic testing will look for changes in the *TPMT* and *NUDT15* genes.

Imaging tests

Imaging scans take pictures of the inside of your child's body to look for cancer. For children with ALL, the images can sometimes provide useful information on where the cancer is and how much of it there is. A radiologist is a doctor who's an expert at reading imaging scans. They will review the images and send the results to your child's care team. These are some of the imaging tests your child may have done:

Chest x-ray

An x-ray uses radiation to take pictures of the inside of the body. Your child may receive a chest x-ray to see if they have a mediastinal mass (a group of abnormal cells). A mediastinal mass forms in the space between the lungs in front of the heart.

CT scan or MRI scan of the head

Your child may need a magnetic resonance imaging (MRI) or computed tomography scan (CT or CAT scan) of their head if they have neurological symptoms. Neurological symptoms, such as headaches, vision changes, tremors, speech difficulties, and a lack of normal facial movement, may be signs that something is affecting how the nervous system functions.

Both types of scans make images of the inside of your child's body. Your child will receive a contrast agent (also called contrast dye) to make the pictures clearer. Contrast is a substance that is injected into a vein and/or mixed with liquid to drink that leaves the body in urine. Tell your child's care team if your child has had allergic reactions to contrast in the past.

CT body scan

A CT scan uses x-rays to take pictures of your child's body from different angles. A computer then combines the pictures to make a 3D image.

MRI and CT scans

MRI and CT scanners look similar, but they're different. Both machines have beds that move into the tunnel-like part of the machine. MRI machines usually have longer and more narrow tunnel spaces.

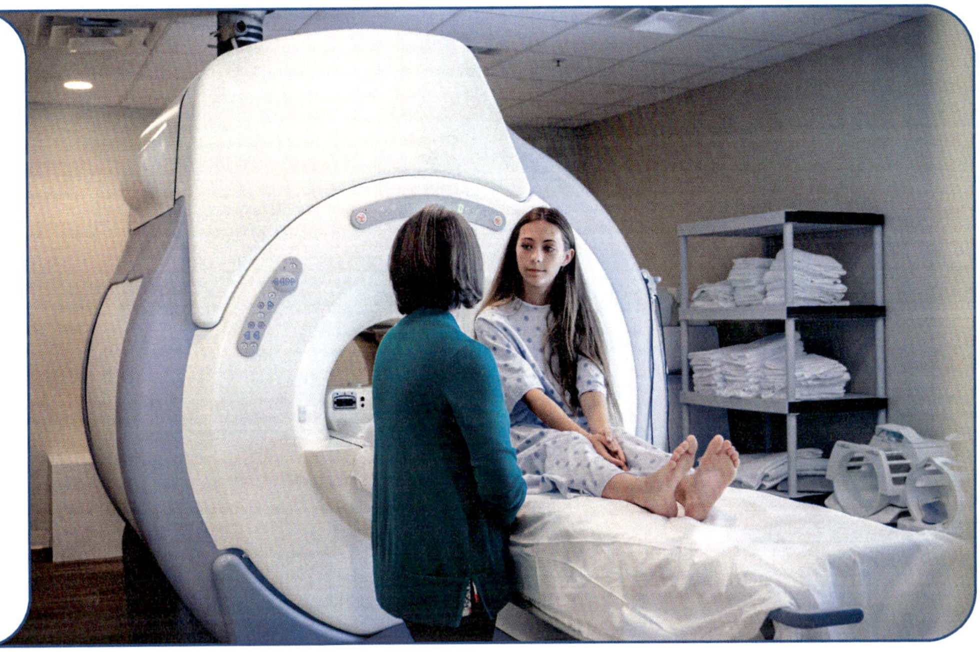

MRI body scan

An MRI scan uses radio waves, powerful magnets, and a computer to take pictures of the inside of the body. MRIs have a tunnel-like design where the magnet surrounds your child.

Whole-body PET scan

A whole-body positron emission tomography (PET) scan is not a common test for ALL, but it may be done in some cases. A PET scan shows whether the cells in your child's body are functioning normally or abnormally. It highlights cells that may be cancerous and can show even small amounts of cancer. A PET scan requires injecting a substance called a radiotracer into your child's bloodstream. The radiotracer is detected during the scan and makes cancer cells appear brighter on the images. Afterward, the radiotracer leaves the body in urine.

More tests and counseling that may be needed before treatment

The additional tests for ALL that your child might need are listed in **Guide 3**, and some are described below.

Heart tests

If your child is going to receive anthracyclines (a type of chemotherapy), they will need to have heart (cardiac) tests done. These tests are used to see how well the heart works. Your child might be referred to a heart specialist called a cardiologist.

Guide 3 Additional tests for ALL your child might need
Testicular exam, including scrotal ultrasound, if needed
CT or MRI scan of the head with contrast, if neurologic symptoms occur
Whole body PET/CT scan, if lymphoblastic lymphoma is suspected
Heart tests for those who will receive certain chemotherapy (anthracyclines)
Infection evaluations, when appropriate
Pregnancy test, if needed, and fertility counseling and fertility preservation, if appropriate
For people who are adolescents and young adults, counseling on stopping smoking, drugs/illicit substances, vaping, and alcohol is encouraged

Watch for infections

When appropriate, testing for infections may also be done. An opportunistic infection is an infection that either happens more often or is more severe because someone's immune system is not working normally. Treatment for ALL can weaken the body's natural defense against infections. Your child will be monitored for opportunistic infections and treated for them, if needed.

Fevers are always considered a medical emergency and your child should be evaluated if they develop one.

Fertility counseling

Fertility counseling is recommended for everyone with pediatric ALL. Some types of treatment can affect fertility, which is the ability to have children. Ask your child's care team how cancer and cancer treatment might change your child's fertility.

More information on fertility and fertility preservation can be found in *NCCN Guidelines for Patients®: Adolescent and Young Adult Cancer*, available at NCCN.org/patientguidelines and on the NCCN Patient Guides for Cancer app.

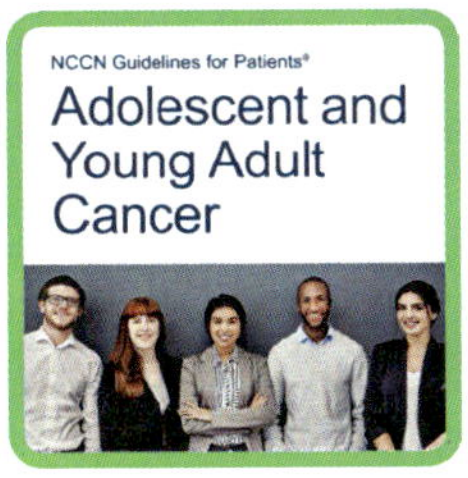

General counseling

Your child's care team will also check on them to see how they're doing emotionally, socially, and mentally. This is called a psychosocial assessment. If your child is a young adult, their care team will also provide counseling on quitting smoking or vaping.

"Have open communication with your child. Remind them that you love them and that they are strong."

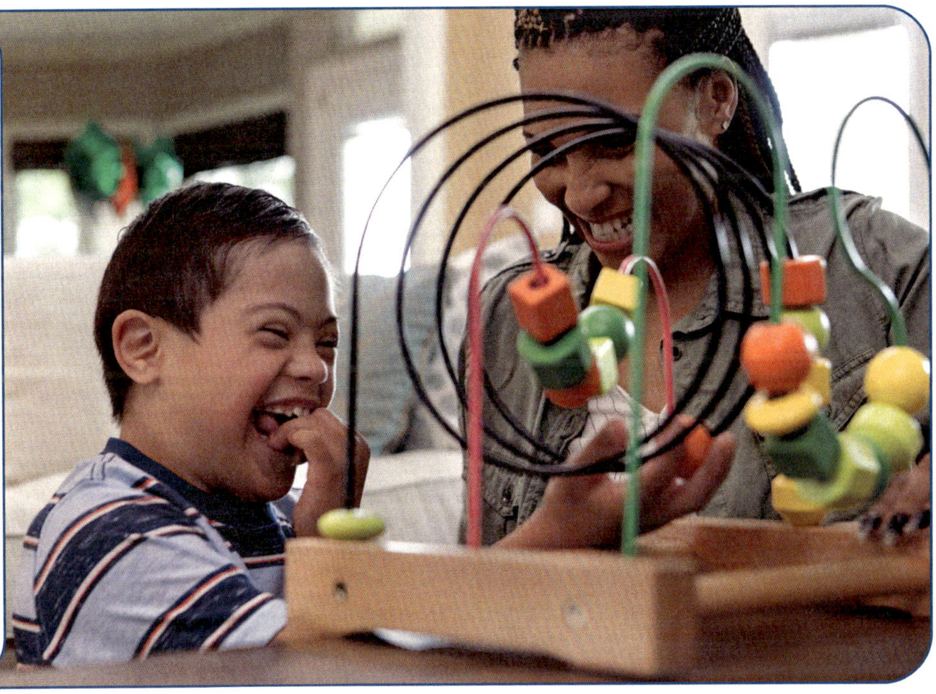

Risk factors

After testing, your child will be placed into a risk group based on the combination of risk factors they have. Risk factors include:

- Age at diagnosis
- White blood cell count at diagnosis
- Certain gene or chromosome mutations, translocations, deletions, and rearrangements
- If leukemia cells are in the brain and spinal fluid (this is called central nervous system involvement) or testicles

Key points

- Imaging tests, a physical exam, and other tests will be done to prepare your child for treatment.
- Leukemia cells can travel to the cerebrospinal fluid that surrounds the spine or brain. A lumbar puncture (spinal tap) will be done to see if cancer is in that area. Acute lymphoblastic leukemia (ALL) can also travel to sites outside of the blood, such as the testicles.
- Blood tests are done to check for signs of disease, and they can help show how well organs are working.
- Your child will get a central venous access device, which allows their care team to give them fluids, blood products, medication, and more.
- Counseling will be offered and can help your child before, during, and after treatment.

Questions to ask

- What tests do you recommend for my child?
- Are the tests done all on the same day? How long will testing take?
- Who will explain the test results to me and when?
- Will my insurance pay for all of the tests?
- Can you explain more about what type of ALL the tests say my child has?

4 Types of treatment

There is more than 1 treatment for acute lymphoblastic leukemia (ALL) in children. This chapter presents an overview of the types of treatment and what to expect. Not everyone will receive the same treatment. However, combination chemotherapy is the standard treatment for pediatric ALL.

All treatment regimens include systemic therapy and/or intrathecal therapy

Systemic therapy is therapy that treats the whole body (such as chemotherapy).

Intrathecal therapy is injected into the cerebrospinal fluid, which surrounds the brain and spine. This allows the therapy to reach these areas, which other treatments can't.

What is systemic therapy?

Systemic therapy is treatment that works throughout the entire body. The therapies travel through the bloodstream to treat cancer cells all over the body. Chemotherapy and targeted therapy are types of systemic therapy.

A treatment **regimen** is a plan for treatment that describes the specific dose, schedule, and length of time the therapy or therapies will be given. All treatments listed in this guide are recommended and appropriate. When helpful, NCCN experts also assign a level of preference to their recommendations for systemic therapies:

- **Preferred therapies** have the most evidence they may work better and be safer than other therapies.
- **Other recommended therapies** can provide effective results but may have less evidence, more side effects, or may not work quite as well as preferred therapies.
- **Therapies used in certain cases** work best for individuals with specific cancer features or health circumstances.

Later chapters describe the specific treatments that are recommended for the different subtypes of acute lymphoblastic leukemia (ALL). They will say whether the systemic therapy treatment is a preferred regimen.

Combination chemotherapy

Chemotherapy is the standard treatment for children with ALL. Many chemotherapies will be given together, which is known as multi-drug chemotherapy or a multi-agent chemotherapy regimen.

Chemotherapies are often combined because each chemotherapy works in a different way to kill cancer cells. Chemotherapies can also be combined with other types of treatments (such as targeted therapy).

Importantly, each type of chemotherapy can also cause different side effects. Your child's care team will check on them throughout treatment to help manage any side effects or uncomfortable feelings. Talk to your child's care team about the types of chemotherapy your child is getting, when your child will get them, and what side effects they could have.

The most common chemotherapy drugs used to treat ALL in children are listed in **Guide 4**. Other types of chemotherapy may be used depending on the type of ALL your child has and how it responds to therapy.

Intrathecal chemotherapy

All treatment plans for pediatric ALL include a type of chemotherapy called intrathecal chemotherapy. Intrathecal chemotherapy is injected into your child's spinal fluid even if no leukemia cells were found in the spinal fluid. It's given so the chemotherapy can reach the brain and spinal cord, which not all other standard chemotherapies are able to do. Some treatment plans include intrathecal chemotherapies throughout therapy, and others don't include it in later-phase maintenance therapy. Because this treatment is given to prevent ALL from spreading to the central nervous system (CNS), it's called CNS prophylaxis or prophylactic treatment.

If ALL is found in your child's CNS at the time of diagnosis, they may need more intrathecal chemotherapy or radiation therapy to the brain.

Guide 4
Chemotherapy drugs for pediatric ALL

- Vincristine
- Cyclophosphamide
- Cytarabine
- Mercaptopurine
- Methotrexate
- Daunorubicin
- Doxorubicin
- Nelarabine
- Pegaspargase and Calaspargase
- Thioguanine

Steroids

Steroids help kill ALL cells, and they're an important part of all the pediatric ALL treatment regimens. They're usually combined with chemotherapy as part of the chemotherapy treatment. The steroids your child might receive are listed in **Guide 5**.

Guide 5
Steroids for pediatric ALL

- Dexamethasone
- Prednisone
- Hydrocortisone

Targeted therapy and immunotherapy

Targeted therapy is a type of treatment that targets specific or unique features of cancer cells. There are many different types of targeted therapy, and some targeted therapies are also considered immunotherapies. Immunotherapy is a type of treatment that uses your immune system to find and kill cancer cells.

Guide 6
Targeted therapies for pediatric ALL

Treatments	Is this treatment an immunotherapy?
• Dasatinib (Sprycel)	No
• Imatinib (Gleevec)	No
• Bortezomib (Velcade)	No
• Revumenib (Revuforj)	No
• Venetoclax (Venclexta)	No
• Ruxolitinib (Jakafi)	No
• Blinatumomab (Blincyto)	Yes
• Inotuzumab ozogamicin (Besponsa)	Yes
• Daratumumab (Darzalex)	Yes
• Tisagenlecleucel (Kymriah)	Yes*

*Tisagenlecleucel is a CAR T-cell therapy.

Guide 6 lists the targeted therapy options that are used to treat pediatric ALL and describes which targeted therapies are also immunotherapies. What type of targeted therapy your child gets depends on the genetic changes of your child's ALL cells and what type of ALL they have.

What is a tyrosine kinase inhibitor?

A tyrosine kinase inhibitor (TKI) is a type of targeted therapy that's used to treat certain types of pediatric ALL. Children with certain genetic changes can receive TKIs in combination with other therapies.

Clinical trials

Talk to your child's doctor about whether a clinical trial may make sense for them. Clinical trials offer options that may either be more effective at curing ALL or cause fewer side effects.

A clinical trial is a type of medical research study. After being developed and tested in a lab, potential new ways of fighting cancer need to be studied in people.

If found to be safe and effective in a clinical trial, a drug, device, or treatment approach may be approved by the U.S. FDA.

Everyone with cancer should carefully consider all of the treatment options available for their cancer type, including standard treatments and clinical trials. Talk to your doctor about whether a clinical trial makes sense for your child.

Phases

Most cancer clinical trials focus on treatment and are done in phases.

- **Phase 1** trials study the safety and side effects of an investigational drug or treatment approach.
- **Phase 2** trials study how well the drug or approach works against a specific type of cancer.
- **Phase 3** trials test the drug or approach against a standard treatment. If the results are good, it may be approved by the FDA.
- **Phase 4** trials study the long-term safety and benefit of an FDA-approved treatment.

Who can enroll?

It depends on the clinical trial's rules, called eligibility criteria. The rules may be about age, cancer type and stage, treatment history, or general health. They ensure that participants are alike in specific ways and that the trial is as safe as possible for the participants.

Informed consent

Clinical trials are managed by a research team. This group of experts will review the study with you in detail, including its purpose and the risks and benefits of joining. All of this information is also provided in an informed consent form. Read the form carefully and ask questions before signing it. Take time to discuss it with people you trust. Keep in mind that your child can leave and seek treatment outside of the clinical trial at any time.

Finding a clinical trial

In the United States

NCCN Cancer Centers
NCCN.org/cancercenters

The National Cancer Institute (NCI)
cancer.gov/about-cancer/treatment/clinical-trials/search

Worldwide

The U.S. National Library of Medicine (NLM)
clinicaltrials.gov

Need help finding a clinical trial?

NCI's Cancer Information Service (CIS)
1.800.4.CANCER (1.800.422.6237)
cancer.gov/contact

Will my child get a placebo?

Placebos (inactive versions of real medicines) are almost never used alone in cancer clinical trials. It is common to receive either a placebo with a standard treatment, or a new drug with a standard treatment. You will be informed, verbally and in writing, if a placebo is part of a clinical trial before your child enrolls.

Are clinical trials free?

There is no fee to enroll in a clinical trial. The study sponsor pays for research-related costs, including the study drug. But you may need to pay for other services, like transportation or childcare, due to extra appointments. During the trial, your child will continue to receive standard cancer care. This care is often covered by insurance.

Radiation therapy

Your child might receive radiation therapy directed at their brain (cranial irradiation) if they have leukemia in their CNS. Radiation therapy uses high-energy radiation to kill cancer cells and shrink tumors. It's given over a certain period of time.

Since ALL can sometimes be found in the testicles, radiation therapy might be given to this area. Radiation therapy directed at the testicles may be given if your child has testicular disease at diagnosis that's still there after induction therapy.

Total body irradiation is another type of radiation therapy. It's radiation for the whole body that can be given in certain situations.

Your child's care team

Treating ALL takes a team approach. Your child's team might include the following specialists:

- **A pediatric oncologist**, who is a doctor that diagnoses and treats cancer in children and young adults.
- **A child life specialist**, who is a healthcare provider that helps children during medical experiences. They will help your child understand the cancer diagnosis, help with any discomfort during treatments and appointments, and provide support.
- **Social workers**, who are people that will help your family emotionally and with other needs. Social workers can also help you find resources to pay for treatment and help your child stay connected to school.
- **Nurses**, who are healthcare providers that will help care for your child. Certain nurses will also give your child chemotherapy.
- **Physicians**, who are doctors that will help with testing and treatment. Different types of physicians will give your child the tests they need, such as blood tests and imaging tests.

Hematopoietic cell transplant

A hematopoietic cell transplant replaces blood-producing (hematopoietic) stem cells that have been destroyed by high doses of chemotherapy or radiation therapy.

You might hear a hematopoietic cell transplant called a stem cell transplant or a bone marrow transplant. This guide will refer to the transplant as a hematopoietic cell transplant. Hematopoietic cell transplants are intense treatments done in specialized centers.

If your child needs a hematopoietic cell transplant, the type they will receive is called an allogeneic hematopoietic cell transplant. This treatment is given if the cancer has not responded well to other treatments or if it was in complete remission and then came back.

Allogeneic hematopoietic cell transplant

An allogeneic transplant uses healthy stem cells from another person (donor) to regrow your child's bone marrow. First, your child will receive treatment with chemotherapy and/or radiation therapy to kill any cancer cells. Next, they will receive an infusion of healthy stem cells from a donor. These cells will form new, healthy bone marrow, which will make healthy blood cells.

Possible side effects

After an allogeneic transplant, there is a chance that the donor cells could react against your child's cells (this is known as graft-versus-host disease, or GVHD). The possibility of GVHD should be discussed with your child's care team, and GVHD can be managed with their transplant team. Your child's care team will also monitor them for infections and other side effects.

More information on GVHD can be found in *NCCN Guidelines for Patients: Graft-Versus-Host Disease*, available at NCCN.org/patientguidelines and on the NCCN Patient Guides for Cancer app.

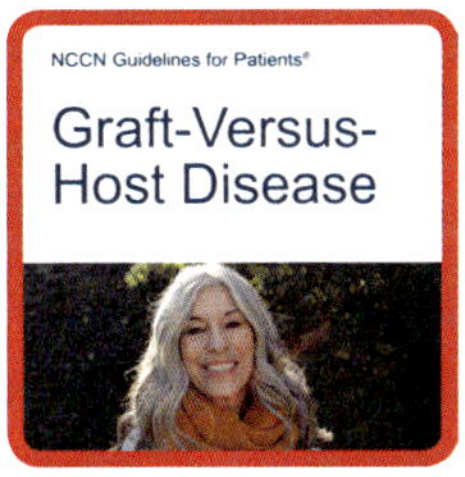

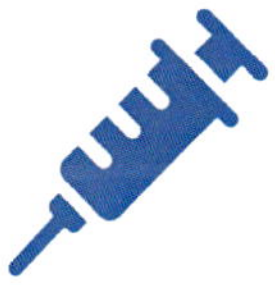

Hematopoietic cell transplant

A hematopoietic cell transplant is a procedure that replaces damaged or destroyed stem cells with healthy stem cells. The healthy stem cells help grow new blood cells.

This transplant is an intense treatment. Because of this, your child will get a particular type of hematopoietic cell transplant known as an allogeneic hematopoietic cell transplant. An allogeneic transplant uses healthy blood stem cells from someone else (a donor) to regrow your child's bone marrow.

Key points

- Combinations of chemotherapy are the main treatment for pediatric acute lymphoblastic leukemia (ALL) treatment. Chemotherapies are often combined with other drug therapies.
- All treatment plans for pediatric ALL include a type of chemotherapy called intrathecal chemotherapy. This is given so the chemotherapy can reach the brain and spinal cord.
- Clinical trials are medical research studies that offer new treatments to people. They offer options that are hopefully more effective at curing ALL or cause fewer side effects. Clinical trials are recommended for children with ALL.
- Targeted therapy focuses on specific or unique features of cancer cells, and many targeted therapies are used to treat pediatric ALL. Some targeted therapies that are available are also immunotherapies (meaning they use the immune system to fight cancer).
- A hematopoietic cell transplant may be a treatment option when the cancer hasn't responded well to treatment or has come back after initially going into remission. This transplant replaces damaged stem cells in the bone marrow with healthy stem cells.

Questions to ask

- Which treatment(s) do you recommend and why?
- What clinical trial options are available?
- What side effects can we expect from treatment?
- How will you treat side effects? What should we look for?
- Are there resources to help pay for treatment or other care my child may need?

5

Phases of treatment

Your child will be given treatment over different time periods or phases. The first phase of treatment is called induction therapy. There are 3 main phases of treatment: induction therapy, consolidation therapy, and maintenance therapy.

What are the different phases of treatment?

The 3 main phases of treatment for pediatric acute lymphoblastic leukemia (ALL) are:

- Induction therapy
- Consolidation therapy
- Maintenance therapy

Importantly, not all doctors use the same terms when discussing treatment.

The number of treatment phases and the type of chemotherapy that your child receives depends on the type of ALL they have and how the first phases of treatment worked.

Induction therapy

Induction therapy is the first phase of treatment. Treatment is a combination of chemotherapies (called multi-drug chemotherapy). Your child will likely spend time in the hospital for part of this treatment.

After induction therapy, your child's care team will check to see how the cancer responded to treatment by doing another bone marrow test. The **treatment regimen** (treatment plan) they receive for consolidation therapy may depend on if the cancer is in complete remission.

Main phases of pediatric ALL treatment

1. **Induction therapy**

The first phase of treatment. Induction therapy is done to kill as many cancer cells as possible. The goal of induction therapy is for ALL to go into **remission** (cancer is in remission when the signs and symptoms of cancer decrease or disappear).

2. **Consolidation therapy**

The second phase of treatment. This is sometimes called intensification therapy. Consolidation therapy is continued treatment given to kill more cancer cells.

3. **Maintenance therapy**

The last phase of treatment, which is usually the longest. The goal of maintenance therapy is to get rid of all the leukemia in the body.

Looking for any leftover cancer cells after treatment

Sensitive lab tests can be used to measure the number of leukemia cells that might be left over after treatment. This is known as looking for minimal residual disease (MRD). Minimal residual disease is the very small number of cancer cells that are left in the body during or after cancer treatment. Not all minimal residual disease can be found with tests though, which means there may still be left-over leukemia cells even if the test shows a negative result.

Throughout the rest of treatment, labs tests will be monitored to see how the cancer is responding to therapy.

Consolidation therapy

After induction therapy, your child will receive another phase of chemotherapy treatment to get rid of any leukemia cells that might still be there. Based on their type of cancer, they might also receive immunotherapy, which uses the body's own immune system to kill cancer cells. The time spent in this or any other phase of treatment can vary. Treatments are based on factors such as age, how the ALL responds to treatment, and any risk factors.

Maintenance therapy

Maintenance therapy, which is sometimes called continuation therapy, is the final and longest stage of treatment for pediatric ALL. Treatment is less intense than prior chemotherapy but is very important for long-term cure of your child's ALL.

"Do not forget to take care of yourself while taking care of your child. It is easy to be completely immersed in their care and not do anything for yourself. Make time for yourself, when possible. It's healthy and will allow you to be strong for your child."

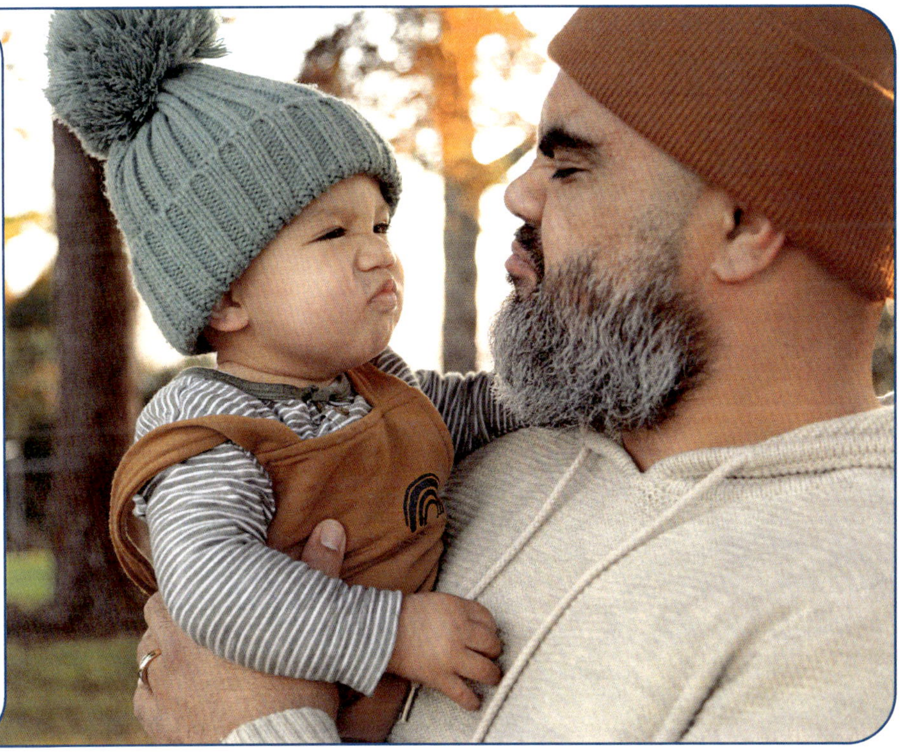

Watching and monitoring time period

The watching and monitoring time period is when your child's care team will check for any changes in your child's condition after treatment is completed. This time period is also called **surveillance**. Your child's care team will monitor for cancer and any side effects.

Types of responses to treatment

After treatment is given, your child's care team will check to see how the cancer responded to treatment. The cancer may:

- Be in remission (cancer went away)
- Have relapsed (cancer went away but then came back)
- Be refractory (cancer did not get better after induction therapy)
- Be progressing (cancer grew or spread)

Remission

Remission is when the symptoms of a disease, such as cancer, decrease or go away. Remission can be short-term (temporary) or long-lasting (permanent).

Partial remission means the signs and symptoms of cancer have decreased after treatment. Complete remission means all signs and symptoms of cancer have gone away.

When a complete remission happens, all of the following are true:

- There are no signs and symptoms of cancer outside of the bone marrow (your child does not have swollen lymph nodes; a swollen spleen; or cancer involving the skin, gums, testicles, and central nervous system)
- No lymphoblasts are found in the blood
- There are a very small number of lymphoblasts found in the bone marrow (less than 5 lymphoblasts out of every 100 blood cells, or 5%)
- Blood cell counts have recovered
- Cancer has not returned in 4 weeks

Progressive disease

When the number of lymphoblasts increases in your child's blood or bone marrow during treatment, it's called progressive disease. ALL is considered progressive when the cancer spreads to other areas or when the number of blasts in the blood or bone marrow increases by at least 25%.

Key points

- There are 3 main phases of treatment for ALL: induction therapy, consolidation therapy, and maintenance therapy.
- Your child's care team will check on them during and between phases of treatment to see how the cancer is responding to treatment.
- Induction therapy is the first phase of treatment. Treatment is a combination of chemotherapies.
- After induction therapy, your child will move onto the consolidation phase. The goal of this phase of treatment is to get rid of any remaining leukemia cells.
- Maintenance, or continuation, therapy is very important and is the final and longest stage of treatment in pediatric ALL.
- The surveillance and monitoring time period is when your child's care team will check for any changes in your child's condition after therapy is complete.
- After treatment, cancer can be in remission (cancer went away), relapsed (cancer went away but then came back), refractory (cancer did not get better after induction therapy), or progressing (cancer grew or spread).

Questions to ask

- How long will my child receive induction therapy for?
- How long will it take to do the tests in between phases of treatment?
- What treatments are done in the hospital? Can any treatments be done at home?
- Who will be my point of contact during each phase of treatment?
- How long is treatment overall?

What's next?

Treatment options for ALL are based on what type of ALL your child has, if the cancer is standard risk or high risk, and if they have the *BCR::ABL1*-positive or *BCR::ABL1*-negative B-ALL. Later treatments are based on their response to the first treatment—this is figured out by something called minimal residual disease (MRD). MRD is the small amount of measurable cancer cells left in the body after treatment.

6

Treatments for *BCR::ABL1*-negative or *BCR::ABL1*-like B-ALL

This chapter explains the treatments for children with *BCR::ABL1*-negative or *BCR::ABL1*-like B-cell acute lymphoblastic leukemia (B-ALL). With this type of cancer, the *BCR::ABL1* gene is not found. It's important to know if your child has this gene or not because it will determine what treatment they get.

How is *BCR::ABL1*-negative B-ALL treated?

The treatment your child receives is based on whether they have standard-risk or high-risk acute lymphoblastic leukemia (ALL). To figure out if the ALL is standard or high risk, your child's care team will look at their white blood cell count and their age at diagnosis. Other features might impact risk, too. Before starting treatment, your child will be placed into a risk group.

According to the Children's Oncology Group (also called COG):

- Standard-risk ALL includes children with a lower white blood cell count who are between 1 and 10 years of age.
- High-risk ALL includes children who have a higher white blood cell count and children who are 10 years of age and over. Having testicular disease, central nervous system disease, or previous treatment with steroids are also considered high risk.

People in the same risk group will likely respond to treatment in the same way. As a result, doctors often use risk groups to help plan treatment.

First treatment: Induction therapy

For children in both risk groups with *BCR::ABL1*-negative or *BCR::ABL1*-like B-cell ALL (B-ALL), treatment options are similar. The preferred treatment option for induction therapy is a clinical trial. If one is not available or if you prefer your child isn't treated in a clinical trial, a standard chemotherapy regimen will be used. **Guide 7** shows these induction therapy options.

Children will get different combinations of chemotherapy depending on their risk group. Importantly, all induction therapy regimens include a combination of chemotherapies. There are many different treatment regimen options for ALL.

After induction therapy is complete, your child's care team will check to see how the cancer responded to treatment. The goal of

Guide 7
Induction therapy options for *BCR::ABL1*-negative or *BCR::ABL1*-like B-ALL

- Clinical trial (preferred)
- Chemotherapy regimen

induction therapy is for the cancer to go into complete remission. After figuring out if a complete remission has happened, your child will start the next phase of treatment, which is consolidation therapy. *Chapter 5: Phases of treatment* explains more about the different responses to treatment.

Second treatment: Consolidation therapy

The consolidation therapy your child gets depends on if the cancer is in complete remission after induction therapy.

Consolidation therapy options if the cancer is in complete remission after induction therapy

Guide 8 describes the treatment options for when ALL is in complete remission after induction therapy.

To better understand how the leukemia has responded to induction therapy, many teams also do a minimal residual disease (MRD) test when checking for remission. This test can detect much lower levels of leukemia cells than the test for complete remission. If no MRD is found (no cancer cells are found after treatment), your child's care team will describe the cancer as being MRD negative. If MRD is found (cancer cells are found after treatment), it's called MRD-positive cancer.

Guide 8
Consolidation therapy options if *BCR::ABL1*-negative or *BCR::ABL1*-like B-ALL is in complete remission after induction therapy

Tests show there are no cancer cells left (MRD-negative result)	• Continue treatment plus blinatumomab				
Tests show there are cancer cells left (MRD-positive result)	• Clinical trial (preferred) • Intensified chemotherapy regimen plus blinatumomab	→	Your child's care team will check to see how the cancer responded to treatment (MRD test)	→	• If the test shows an MRD-negative result, treatment is chemotherapy and blinatumomab • If tests show an MRD-positive result, treatment options are a clinical trial (preferred), chemotherapy regimen, and blinatumomab

Consolidation therapy options if the cancer isn't in complete remission after induction therapy

If induction therapy did not result in a complete remission, your child's care team will give them more treatment. Cancer that did not respond to treatment is known as refractory cancer. **Guide 9** describes treatment options for this type of cancer.

> "Get organized! Write things down and review them so that you understand all the care that your child is receiving. This will also be a good way to come up with questions."

Guide 9
Treatment options for refractory *BCR::ABL1*-negative or *BCR::ABL1*-like B-ALL

Treatment		Consolidation therapy
• Clinical trial (preferred) • Systemic therapy • Blinatumomab • Tisagenlecleucel • Inotuzumab ozogamicin	→ Your child's care team will check to see how the cancer responded to treatment →	• If a complete remission happens: Hematopoietic cell transplant • Different therapy or best supportive care

Third treatment: Maintenance therapy

Your child will receive maintenance therapy after the consolidation phase of treatment. This is usually the longest phase of therapy and is less intense than previous phases.

If the cancer is in remission, then maintenance chemotherapy will be given. A hematopoietic cell transplant is an option in some cases, too (**Guide 10**).

If the cancer is not in complete remission, your child will be treated for refractory cancer. **Guide 9** on page 39 describes these treatment options.

After maintenance therapy: Surveillance and monitoring

After maintenance therapy or a transplant, if the cancer is in complete remission your child will be monitored and enter the surveillance phase of treatment. This is described in **Guide 11**.

Guide 10
Maintenance therapy options for *BCR::ABL1*-negative or *BCR::ABL1*-like B-ALL

- Chemotherapy regimen
- Hematopoietic cell transplant (for children with cancer that was not in complete remission after induction therapy)

It's very important for your child to continue taking their medicine as prescribed without missing or skipping doses. This helps prevent a relapse.

If cancer comes back after a complete remission

If your child's cancer comes back after a period of remission, this is known as a relapse. The goal of treatment after a relapse is to achieve remission again.

Treatment options are based on the amount of time from diagnosis to relapse. Treatments are also based on if cancer is found in bone marrow (isolated medullary relapse), areas other than the bone marrow (isolated extramedullary relapse), or in the bone marrow and other areas (combined relapse).

After your child receives testing for the *BCR::ABL1* gene to make sure they still have *BCR::ABL1*-negative or *BCR::ABL1*-like B-ALL, they will receive treatment. Most treatment plans for relapsed cancer eventually lead to a hematopoietic cell transplant.

Guide 11
Surveillance and monitoring for ALL

Surveillance	1 year after treatment	➞	Every 1 to 4 months your child will get a: • Physical exam and testicular exam • Complete blood count (CBC) with differential • Liver function test until levels are normal
	2 years after treatment	➞	Every 2 to 6 months your child will get a: • Physical exam and testicular exam • CBC with differential
	3 years after treatment	➞	Every 6 to 12 months, or as needed, your child will get a: • Physical exam and testicular exam • CBC with differential
Additional tests	• Bone marrow aspiration and cerebrospinal fluid testing, if your child's care team thinks the cancer might have come back		
Monitoring for late side effects	• Echocardiogram (heart test) if needed • Neuropsychological testing if needed to check for neurologic issues • Weight monitoring (people with a history of childhood ALL are at increased risk of developing obesity) • See *Long-Term Follow-up Guidelines for Survivors of Childhood, Adolescent, and Young Adult Cancers* from the Children's Oncology Group (COG) at survivorshipguidelines.org • See *NCCN Guidelines for Patients: Adolescent and Young Adult Cancer* at NCCN.org/patientguidelines.		

Treatment options for first relapses

Treatment options for first relapses that either happened early or later on are a clinical trial (preferred) or systemic therapy. After these treatments, your child's care team will check to see how the cancer responded to treatment. Then, consolidation therapy will be given. See **Guide 12** for information on what treatments are given after the first relapse.

Treatment options when a first relapse happens after a hematopoietic cell transplant

Treatment options for a relapse that happens after a hematopoietic cell transplant are:

- Clinical trial (preferred)
- Systemic therapy
- Blinatumomab
- Tisagenlecleucel (CAR T-cell therapy)
- Inotuzumab ozogamicin

Guide 12
Treatment options for first relapses: *BCR::ABL1*-negative or *BCR::ABL1*-like B-ALL

Response after treatment with a clinical trial or systemic therapy:	Consolidation therapy		
ALL is in complete remission and tests show an MRD-negative result	• Clinical trial (preferred) • Chemotherapy • Blinatumomab	→	• If early first relapse: Hematopoietic cell transplant • If late first relapse: Maintenance chemotherapy or consider hematopoietic cell transplant
ALL is in complete remission but tests show an MRD-positive result	• Clinical trial (preferred) • Chemotherapy • Blinatumomab • Tisagenlecleucel • Inotuzumab ozogamicin	→	• Hematopoietic cell transplant
ALL is not in complete remission	• Clinical trial (preferred) • Systemic therapy • Blinatumomab • Tisagenlecleucel • Inotuzumab ozogamicin	→	• If a complete remission occurs: Hematopoietic cell transplant • If a complete remission does not occur: Different therapy or best supportive care

Your child's care team will check to see how the cancer responded to the treatment and then they'll get consolidation therapy.

- If the cancer is in complete remission, then your child could be given a second hematopoietic cell transplant.
- If the cancer is not in complete remission, then treatment will be one of the options listed in the next section.

If cancer doesn't respond to treatment or comes back more than once

Treatment options for multiple relapses are the same as those for refractory cancer (**Guide 9** on page 39). These options include:

- Clinical trial (preferred)
- Systemic therapy
- Blinatumomab
- Tisagenlecleucel (CAR T-cell therapy)
- Inotuzumab ozogamicin

Before starting consolidation therapy, your child's care team will check to see how the cancer responded to treatment.

- If the cancer is in complete remission, they will get a hematopoietic cell transplant.
- If the cancer is not in complete remission, then treatment might be another therapy or supportive care.

Key points

- *BCR::ABL1*-negative and *BCR::ABL1*-like B-cell acute lymphoblastic leukemia (B-ALL) are types of B-ALL where the *BCR::ABL1* gene is not found.
- Induction therapy is the first phase of treatment, which can be given with a clinical trial (preferred) or a chemotherapy regimen.
- The consolidation therapy your child gets depends on if the cancer is in complete remission after induction therapy.
- If the cancer is not in complete remission after consolidation therapy, your child will receive treatment for refractory cancer.
- If the cancer is in complete remission after consolidation therapy, your child will receive maintenance therapy.
- There are treatment options if the cancer comes back (relapses).

Questions to ask

- How does my child's risk group affect the treatment options?
- Does the order of treatments matter?
- What should I do if my child misses or skips a dose of treatment?
- Why is a clinical trial the preferred option for this type of B-ALL?
- What services are available to help us through this stressful time?

7

Treatments for *BCR::ABL1*-positive B-ALL

BCR::ABL1-positive B-cell acute lymphoblastic leukemia (B-ALL) is when the cancer has the *BCR::ABL1* gene. Treatment is usually a combination of chemotherapies and a tyrosine kinase inhibitor (TKI), which is a type of targeted therapy.

What treatments are given for *BCR::ABL1*-positive B-ALL?

Treatment for *BCR::ABL1*-positive B-cell acute lymphoblastic leukemia (B-ALL) is usually a combination of therapies that includes targeted therapies (typically tyrosine kinase inhibitors, also known as TKIs) and chemotherapies. Treatment can be done as part of a clinical trial, which is preferred when available, or as part of standard cancer care.

First treatment: Induction therapy

Induction therapy is a combination of therapies. The preferred treatment option is a clinical trial including a TKI, but a chemotherapy regimen plus a TKI can also be given (**Guide 13**).

The TKIs that your child could receive as part of their treatment regimen are:

- Imatinib (Gleevec)
- Dasatinib (Sprycel)

After induction therapy is complete, your child's care team will check to see how the cancer responded to treatment (see *Chapter 5: Phases of treatment* for more information on responses to treatment). Tests will look for minimal residual disease (MRD), which is when a small number of cancer cells are left in the body during or after treatment. When no MRD is found, your child's care team will describe the cancer as being MRD negative. When MRD is found, it's called MRD-positive cancer. After your child's care team figures out how the cancer responded to treatment, your child will start the next phase of treatment.

Second treatment: Consolidation therapy

Before starting the consolidation phase of treatment, your child will be placed into a risk group. Risk is based on many different factors, including how much MRD is left after induction therapy. A risk group will determine what treatment has the best chance of helping the cancer go into remission.

Guide 13
Induction therapy options for *BCR::ABL1*-positive B-ALL

- Clinical trial plus a TKI (preferred)
- Chemotherapy regimen plus a TKI

If the tests show that there is very little cancer left (low levels of MRD), your child is considered to have standard-risk disease and will receive:

- Chemotherapy plus blinatumomab and a TKI

If there are still cancer cells found (MRD is positive) and the cancer is not in complete remission, then it's considered high risk. The treatment options include:

- Clinical trial (preferred)
- Chemotherapy plus blinatumomab and a TKI
- Blinatumomab and a TKI

Third treatment: Maintenance therapy

Maintenance therapy is given after the consolidation phase of treatment. This is usually the longest phase of therapy and is less intense than the other phases. Maintenance therapy depends on if your child is in the standard-risk or high-risk group.

Treatment options for children with standard-risk ALL are:

- Systemic therapy plus a TKI
- Hematopoietic cell transplant

Treatment options for children with high-risk ALL are:

- Hematopoietic cell transplant
  - After hematopoietic cell transplant, a TKI may be given

After maintenance therapy: Surveillance and monitoring

After maintenance therapy or a transplant, if the cancer is in complete remission your child will be monitored and enter the surveillance phase of treatment (described in **Guide 14**).

> **"Come to each and every appointment with all of your questions and concerns and do not leave until you get them all answered."**

Guide 14
Surveillance and monitoring for ALL

Surveillance	1 year after treatment →	Every 1 to 4 months your child will get a: • Physical exam and testicular exam • Complete blood count (CBC) with differential • Liver function test until levels are normal
	2 years after treatment →	Every 2 to 6 months your child will get a: • Physical exam and testicular exam • CBC with differential
	3 years after treatment →	Every 6 to 12 months, or as needed, your child will get a: • Physical exam and testicular exam • CBC with differential
Additional tests	• Bone marrow aspiration and cerebrospinal fluid testing, if your child's care team thinks the cancer might have come back	
Monitoring for late side effects	• Echocardiogram (heart test) if needed • Neuropsychological testing if needed to check for neurologic issues • Weight monitoring (people with a history of childhood ALL are at increased risk of developing obesity) • See *Long-Term Follow-up Guidelines for Survivors of Childhood, Adolescent, and Young Adult Cancers* from the Children's Oncology Group (COG) at survivorshipguidelines.org • See *NCCN Guidelines for Patients: Adolescent and Young Adult Cancer* at NCCN.org/patientguidelines.	

If the cancer is not in complete remission, your child will receive treatment for refractory disease. **Guide 15** details therapies for refractory cancer.

If cancer comes back after a complete remission

If the cancer comes back after a period of remission, this is known as a relapse. The goal of treatment after a relapse is to achieve remission again. Treatment options are based on the amount of time from diagnosis to relapse. Treatments are also based on if cancer is found in bone marrow (isolated medullary relapse), areas other than the bone marrow (isolated extramedullary relapse), or in the bone marrow and other areas (combined relapse).

It's very important for your child to continue taking their medicine as prescribed without missing or skipping doses. This helps prevent a relapse.

After your child receives testing for the *BCR::ABL1* gene to make sure they still have *BCR::ABL1*-positive B-ALL, they will receive treatment. Most treatment plans for relapsed cancer eventually lead to a hematopoietic cell transplant.

Guide 15
Treatment options for refractory *BCR::ABL1*-positive B-ALL

Treatment				Consolidation therapy
• Clinical trial (preferred) • Systemic therapy • Blinatumomab • Tisagenlecleucel • Inotuzumab ozogamicin	→	Your child's care team will check to see how the cancer responded to treatment	→	• If a complete remission happens: Hematopoietic cell transplant • If a complete remission doesn't happen: Different therapy or best supportive care

Treatment options for first relapses

Treatment options for first relapses that either happened early or later on are a clinical trial (preferred) or systemic therapy. After these treatments, your child's care team will check to see how the cancer responded to treatment. Then, consolidation therapy will be given. See **Guide 16** for information on what treatments are given after the first relapse.

Guide 16
Treatment options for first relapses: *BCR::ABL1*-positive B-ALL

Response after treatment with a clinical trial or systemic therapy:			Consolidation therapy
ALL is in complete remission and tests show an MRD-negative result	• Clinical trial (preferred) • Chemotherapy • Blinatumomab	→	• If early first relapse: Hematopoietic cell transplant • If late first relapse: Maintenance chemotherapy, or consider hematopoietic cell transplant
ALL is in complete remission but tests show an MRD-positive result	• Clinical trial (preferred) • Chemotherapy • Blinatumomab • Tisagenlecleucel • Inotuzumab ozogamicin	→	• Hematopoietic cell transplant
ALL is not in complete remission	• Clinical trial (preferred) • Systemic therapy • Blinatumomab • Tisagenlecleucel • Inotuzumab ozogamicin	→	• If a complete remission occurs: hematopoietic cell transplant • If a complete remission does not occur: Different therapy or best supportive care

Treatment options when a first relapse happens after a hematopoietic cell transplant

Treatment options for a relapse that happens after a hematopoietic cell transplant are:

- Clinical trial (preferred)
- Systemic therapy
- Blinatumomab
- Tisagenlecleucel (CAR-T cell therapy)
- Inotuzumab ozogamicin

Your child's care team will check to see how the cancer responded to the treatment and then they'll get consolidation therapy.

- If the cancer is in complete remission, then your child could be given a second hematopoietic cell transplant
- If the cancer is not in complete remission, then treatment will be one of the options listed in the next section

If cancer doesn't respond to treatment or comes back more than once

Treatment options for multiple relapses are the same as those for refractory cancer (**Guide 15**). These options include:

- Clinical trial (preferred)
- Systemic therapy
- Blinatumomab
- Tisagenlecleucel (CAR T-cell therapy)
- Inotuzumab ozogamicin

Before starting consolidation therapy, your child's care team will check to see how the cancer responded to treatment.

- If the cancer is in complete remission, they will get a hematopoietic cell transplant
- If the cancer is not in complete remission, then treatment might be another therapy or supportive care

Key points

- *BCR::ABL1*-positive B-cell acute lymphoblastic leukemia (B-ALL) is B-ALL where the BCR::ABL1 gene is found in the leukemia cells.
- Treatment is usually a combination of systemic therapies, including a type of targeted therapy called a tyrosine kinase inhibitor (TKI).
- Induction therapy is a clinical trial plus a TKI (preferred) or a chemotherapy regimen plus a TKI. TKI options are imatinib and dasatinib.
- Before starting the consolidation phase of treatment, your child will be placed into a risk group. Consolidation therapies are different for children in different risk groups.
- If the cancer is not in complete remission after consolidation therapy, your child will receive treatment for refractory cancer.
- If the cancer is in complete remission after consolidation therapy, your child will receive maintenance therapy.
- There are more treatment options if the cancer comes back (relapses).

Questions to ask

- How can I prepare my child for treatment?
- Does the order of treatments matter?
- What should I do if my child misses or skips a dose?
- Why is a clinical trial plus a TKI the preferred option for this type of B-ALL?
- What services are available to help us through this stressful time?

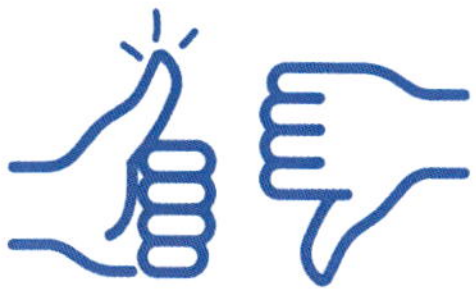

Let us know what you think!

Please take a moment to complete an online survey about the NCCN Guidelines for Patients.
NCCN.org/patients/response

8

Treatments for T-ALL

T-cell acute lymphoblastic leukemia (T-ALL) is a type of ALL that starts in T-cell lymphocytes. Treatment options include a clinical trial or chemotherapy regimen. Other systemic therapies might be given, too.

How is T-ALL treated?

T-cell acute lymphoblastic leukemia (T-ALL) is usually treated with chemotherapy regimens. Some people may receive a hematopoietic cell transplant. Clinical trials are also an option.

First treatment: Induction therapy

First, your child will receive induction therapy. A clinical trial is the preferred treatment option for induction therapy. If a clinical trial is not available, your child will be treated with a chemotherapy regimen. After induction therapy, your child's care team will check to see how the cancer responded to treatment.

Second treatment: Consolidation therapy

Your child will continue receiving chemotherapy for the consolidation therapy part of treatment.

After they finish consolidation therapy, their care team will check again to see how the cancer responded to treatment.

Third treatment: Maintenance (or continuation) therapy

After completing consolidation therapy, your child's care team will determine what the next best step of treatment is.

If the cancer is in complete remission after consolidation therapy

If your child completes consolidation therapy and the cancer is in complete remission, they will receive more treatment. Their care team will determine if the cancer is standard risk, high risk, or very high risk. The next treatment they receive depends on what risk the cancer is.

- Children with standard- or high-risk cancer will continue receiving chemotherapy.
- Children with very high-risk cancer will receive treatment in a clinical trial (preferred), continue chemotherapy, or get another treatment. Afterward, a hematopoietic cell transplant may be given.

Your child will then move on to the surveillance and monitoring phase of treatment where their care team will check on them.

Treatments for T-ALL

Induction therapy:

- Clinical trial (preferred)
- Chemotherapy regimen

Your child's care team will check to see how the cancer responded to treatment

Consolidation therapy:

- Continue chemotherapy

Your child's care team will check to see how the cancer responded to treatment

If the cancer is in complete remission:

For children with very high-risk ALL:

Maintenance therapy options:

- Clinical trial (preferred)
- Continue chemotherapy regimen
- Different therapy
- Consider a hematopoietic cell transplant after 1 of the 3 continued treatments above are given

For children with standard- or high-risk ALL

Maintenance therapy options:

- Continue chemotherapy regimen

If the cancer isn't in complete remission after consolidation therapy

If your child completes consolidation therapy and the cancer is not in remission, they will receive treatment in a clinical trial (preferred) or systemic therapy. Afterward, their care team will see how the cancer responded to the treatment.

- If the cancer is in complete remission, they'll receive more treatment in a clinical trial (preferred) or will get a chemotherapy regimen. In uncommon cases, a hematopoietic cell transplant can be given after this treatment, too.
- If the cancer is not in remission, they'll receive treatment in a clinical trial (preferred) or will get systemic therapy. After treatment is given, your child's care team will check again to see how the cancer responded to treatment. If it's in complete remission, they'll get a hematopoietic cell transplant. If it's not in complete remission, they'll get another treatment or supportive care.

Surveillance and monitoring

After maintenance therapy or a hematopoietic cell transplant, if the cancer is in complete remission your child will be monitored and enter the surveillance phase of treatment. **Guide 17** describes how the surveillance and monitoring process works.

It's very important for your child to continue taking their medicine as prescribed without missing or skipping doses. This helps prevent a relapse.

If cancer comes back after a complete remission

If the cancer comes back after a complete remission, your child can receive more treatment. Options include a clinical trial (preferred) or systemic therapy. After treatment, their care team will check to see how the cancer responded to treatment. If the cancer is in complete remission, they will receive more treatment with a clinical trial (preferred) or chemotherapy. A hematopoietic cell transplant can be given after these treatments, too.

If the cancer is not in complete remission, your child will get the treatments described in the next section, *If cancer doesn't respond to treatment or comes back more than once.*

Guide 17
Surveillance and monitoring for ALL

Surveillance	1 year after treatment →	Every 1 to 4 months your child will get a: • Physical exam and testicular exam • Complete blood count (CBC) with differential • Liver function test until levels are normal
	2 years after treatment →	Every 2 to 6 months your child will get a: • Physical exam and testicular exam • CBC with differential
	3 years after treatment →	Every 6 to 12 months, or as needed, your child will get a: • Physical exam and testicular exam • CBC with differential
Additional tests	• Bone marrow aspiration and cerebrospinal fluid testing, if your child's care team thinks the cancer might have come back	
Monitoring for late side effects	• Echocardiogram (heart test) if needed • Neuropsychological testing if needed to check for neurologic issues • Weight monitoring (people with a history of childhood ALL are at increased risk of developing obesity) • See *Long-Term Follow-up Guidelines for Survivors of Childhood, Adolescent, and Young Adult Cancers* from the Children's Oncology Group (COG) at survivorshipguidelines.org • See *NCCN Guidelines for Patients: Adolescent and Young Adult Cancer* at NCCN.org/patientguidelines.	

If cancer doesn't respond to treatment or comes back more than once

Treatment options for refractory cancer (cancer that hasn't responded to treatment) are the same as the options for multiple relapses (cancer that's come back after being in complete remission more than once). These options include:

- Clinical trial (preferred)
- Systemic therapy

After this treatment, your child's care team will check to see how the cancer responded to treatment.

- If the cancer is in complete remission, they will get a hematopoietic cell transplant.
- If the cancer is not in complete remission, then treatment might be another therapy or supportive care.

Key points

- T-cell acute lymphoblastic leukemia (T-ALL) is ALL that starts in T-cell lymphocytes.
- Induction therapy is a clinical trial (preferred) or a chemotherapy regimen.
- Consolidation therapy is continuing chemotherapy treatment, and afterward, your child's care team will check to see how the cancer responded to treatment.
- Treatments after consolidation therapy depend on if the cancer is in complete remission. If it's in complete remission, your child will get **maintenance** therapy. If it's not in complete remission, they will receive treatment in a clinical trial (preferred) or systemic therapy.

Questions to ask

- How can I prepare my child for treatment?
- Does the order of treatments matter?
- What should I do if my child misses or skips a dose?
- Why is a clinical trial the preferred option for this type of T-ALL?
- What services are available to help us through this stressful time?

9

Treatments for infant ALL

Treatment for infants (children under 12 months of age) with acute lymphoblastic leukemia (ALL) is different from treatment for older children. Your child's care team will explain all the options to you. It's important to know that treatment is based on if a gene called *KMT2A* is rearranged.

First treatment: Induction therapy

Before your child receives their first treatment, their care team will do a test to see if the *KMT2A* gene is rearranged. There are 2 treatment options for all infants:

- Clinical trial (preferred)
- Interfant induction

Interfant induction is a treatment plan that includes many different therapies. All treatment plans include systemic therapy (works throughout the whole body) and intrathecal therapy (injected into the spinal fluid), which is given to prevent or treat central nervous system disease.

After Interfant induction, the next stage of treatment is consolidation therapy. The type of consolidation therapy your child will receive depends on if the *KMT2A* gene is rearranged.

"It's helpful to hear other people's stories, share information, and to learn about resources available for children with leukemia."

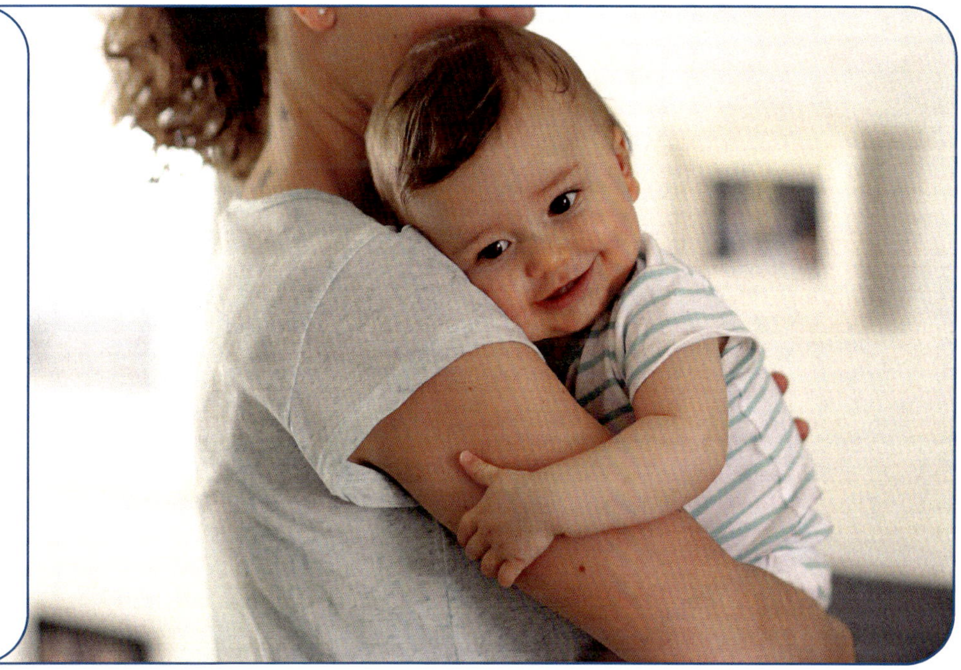

Second treatment: If the *KMT2A* gene is rearranged

If tests show that the *KMT2A* gene is rearranged, your child will get the next phase of treatment (consolidation therapy) with Interfant intensive chemotherapy plus blinatumomab (Blincyto).

After they receive this treatment, they'll move on to the maintenance phase of treatment where they'll get more chemotherapy. Your child's care team may also give them a hematopoietic cell transplant instead of maintenance chemotherapy if the cancer is high risk.

After maintenance chemotherapy or a transplant, your child will enter the monitoring part of treatment. **Guide 18** describes how the surveillance and monitoring process works.

Second treatment: If the *KMT2A* gene is not rearranged

If your child does not have a rearranged *KMT2A* gene, they will get the next phase of treatment (consolidation therapy). They'll be treated with Interfant consolidation therapy plus blinatumomab. Most Interfant consolidation therapy regimens are a combination of chemotherapy drugs and a steroid. Sometimes blinatumomab is added, too. Another option is to receive the same consolidation therapy that children with *BCR::ABL1*-negative or *BCR::ABL1*-like B-ALL get (chemotherapy regimen plus blinatumomab).

After your child receives treatment, they will enter the monitoring part of treatment. **Guide 18** describes how the surveillance and monitoring process works.

Second treatments for infant ALL

If the *KMT2A* gene is rearranged

- Interfant intensive chemotherapy plus blinatumomab

↓

- Chemotherapy
- Hematopoietic cell transplant (if the cancer is high risk)

↓

- Monitoring

If the *KMT2A* gene is not rearranged

- Interfant consolidation therapy plus blinatumomab
- Chemotherapy regimen plus blinatumomab

Guide 18
Surveillance and monitoring for ALL: Checking on your child after treatment

Monitoring (also called surveillance	1 year after treatment →	Every 1 to 4 months your child will get a: • Physical exam and testicular exam • Complete blood count (CBC) with differential • Liver function test until levels are normal
	2 years after treatment →	Every 2 to 6 months your child will get a: • Physical exam and testicular exam • CBC with differential
	3 years after treatment →	Every 6 to 12 months, or as needed, your child will get a: • Physical exam and testicular exam • CBC with differential
Additional tests	• Bone marrow aspiration and cerebrospinal fluid testing, if your child's care team thinks the cancer might have come back	
Monitoring for late side effects	• Echocardiogram (heart test) if needed • Neuropsychological testing if needed to check for neurologic issues • Weight monitoring (people with a history of childhood ALL are at increased risk of developing obesity) • See *Long-Term Follow-up Guidelines for Survivors of Childhood, Adolescent, and Young Adult Cancers* from the Children's Oncology Group (COG) at survivorshipguidelines.org • See *NCCN Guidelines for Patients: Adolescent and Young Adult Cancer* at NCCN.org/patientguidelines.	

Key points

- Infants are children under 12 months of age. Treatment for infants with acute lymphoblastic anemia (ALL) is different from treatment for older children.
- The first treatment your child will get is a clinical trial (preferred) or Interfant induction therapy. Interfant induction therapy is a treatment plan that includes many different therapies.
- The second treatment (consolidation therapy) your child gets depends on if a gene called *KMT2A* is rearranged.
- Treatments are usually a combination of chemotherapies. Sometimes a drug called blinatumomab is given, and a hematopoietic cell transplant is an option for some infants.

Questions to ask

- Does my child have the *KMT2A* gene? What does this mean for treatment options?
- Which treatment do you recommend and why?
- How are treatments going to be given to my child?
- Is a clinical trial an option for my child?
- What services are available to help us through this stressful time?

10
Supportive care

Supportive care is given to improve your child's quality of life. It helps manage the symptoms of acute lymphoblastic leukemia (ALL) and the side effects of treatment. This chapter discusses possible side effects and treatments. Supportive care can also help with other needs, such as paying for care, getting transportation to care, and more.

What is supportive care?

Supportive care is an important part of cancer care. The goal is to improve your child's quality of life during and after cancer treatment. Supportive care is for everyone with cancer and their families, not just for those at the end of life.

Supportive care includes a wide range of services. Supportive care prevents or manages the symptoms of cancer and the side effects of cancer treatment, like pain and cancer-related fatigue. It also addresses the mental, social, emotional, and spiritual concerns faced by people with cancer.

Supportive care provides help with additional needs, such as:

- Making treatment decisions
- Coordinating your care
- Paying for care
- Planning for advance care and end of life

Read more about the types of support you may receive in *NCCN Guidelines for Patients: Palliative Care*, available at NCCN.org/patientguidelines and on the NCCN Patient Guides for Cancer app.

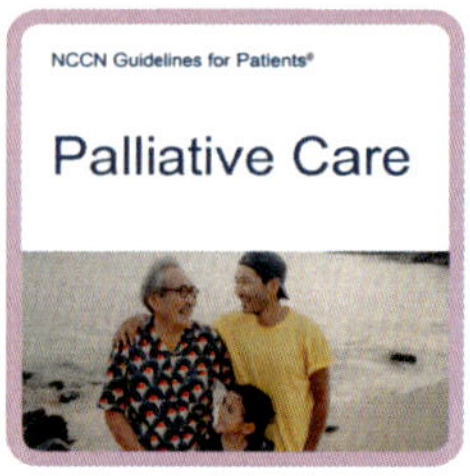

Treatments for common side effects

All cancer treatments can cause unwanted health issues called side effects. The side effects your child experiences depend on many factors, such as the particular treatments they get. Some side effects can be harmful to health while others are just unpleasant. Despite these side effects, the benefits of treatment outweigh the potential risks. Tell your child's care team about any new or worsening symptoms they have.

There are certain side effects of acute lymphoblastic anemia (ALL) treatment that are more common in children. This section explains the common side effects your child may have. The section *Managing the side effects of certain ALL treatments*, on page 67, explains the common side effects of ALL treatments.

Infections

Drug treatment for ALL can weaken the body's natural defense against infections. Infections are more common and more severe in people with a weakened immune system. It's important for infections to be treated early before they get worse.

Your child's care team will monitor their condition and will recommend any vaccines, if needed.

If your child has a fever during therapy, they will need to see a doctor and be treated right away. They'll be given antibiotics, and their care team will check on them.

Preventing infections

If your child's care team thinks they might have low levels of certain white blood cells (neutropenia) at some point during treatment, they may be given an antibiotic to try to prevent a bacterial infection. This is because low levels of these white blood cells can lead to frequent or severe infections.

Children with ALL are also more likely to develop a fungal pneumonia called *Pneumocystis jirovecii*, so your child's care team will give them medicine to help prevent this. The preferred medicine to prevent fungal pneumonia is trimethoprim sulfamethoxazole (Bactrim, Septra, or another agent).

Antifungal medicines may also be recommended during certain phases of treatment.

Tumor lysis syndrome

Tumor lysis syndrome is a serious side effect of cancer treatment. When tumor lysis syndrome happens, the cancer cells that are being killed by treatment fill the bloodstream with toxic substances and substances in blood are not balanced. Sometimes tumor lysis syndrome can even start before treatment begins because leukemia cells are fragile and grow and break apart quickly in the blood.

There are different treatments for tumor lysis syndrome, such as hydration with IV fluids and drug treatments. Treatment depends on what substances are out of balance and how well your child's kidneys are working. Your child's care team will check their labs frequently to make sure the treatment is working the way it's supposed to.

Sore or dry mouth (mucositis)

Mucositis is when certain cells that are inside of the digestive tract, including in the mouth and stomach, become painful, swollen, or irritated. NCCN guidelines recommend that your child see a dentist before they start treatment with chemotherapy.

To prevent mucositis, your child's care team may give them ice chips or cold water when they receive some chemotherapy agents. They may also recommend special rinses or mouthwashes.

Nausea and vomiting

Nausea (an uncomfortable feeling where it feels like you might vomit) and vomiting are common side effects of treatment. Your child will be given medicine to prevent nausea and vomiting.

High blood sugar

One possible side effect of treatment is high blood sugar, which is also called hyperglycemia. If your child has high blood sugar, insulin can be given to lower blood sugar levels.

Fatigue

Fatigue is extreme tiredness and inability to function due to lack of energy. Fatigue may be caused by cancer, or it may be a side effect of treatment. Let your child's care team know how your child is feeling and if fatigue is getting in the way of them doing the things they enjoy.

Organ issues

Treatment might cause your child's kidneys, liver, heart, and pancreas not to work as well as they should. Your child's care team will regularly check on their organs and run tests to make sure treatment is not harming any major organs.

Neurotoxicity

Some treatments can damage the nervous system (neurotoxicity), causing problems with concentration; memory; and other issues, such as dizziness and headaches. Although rare, seizures and confusion can also occur. If your child's ALL treatment includes the chemotherapy methotrexate or the CAR T-cell therapy tisagenlecleucel (Kymriah), then they will be monitored for neurotoxicity.

More information on supportive care is available at NCCN.org/patientguidelines and on the NCCN Patient Guides for Cancer app.

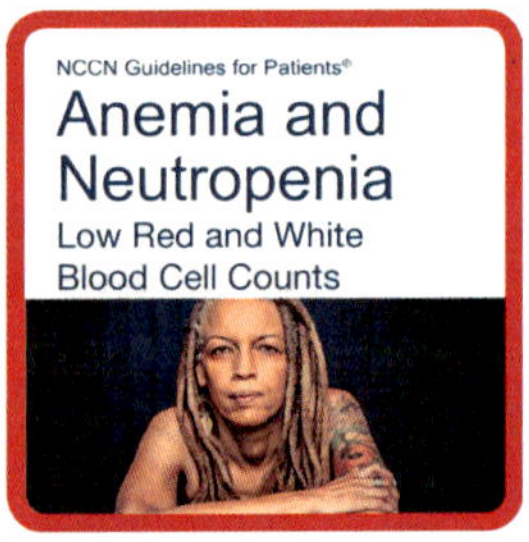

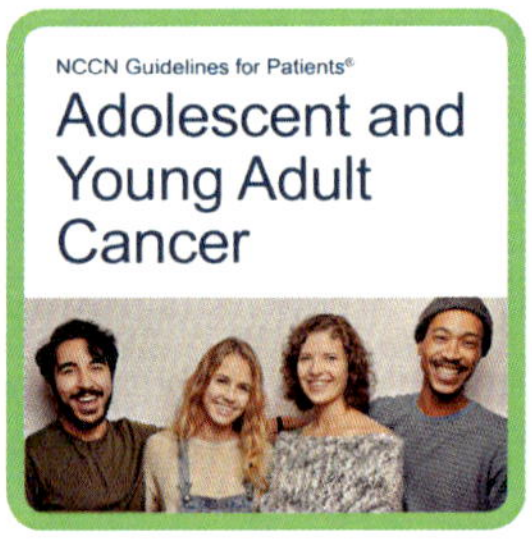

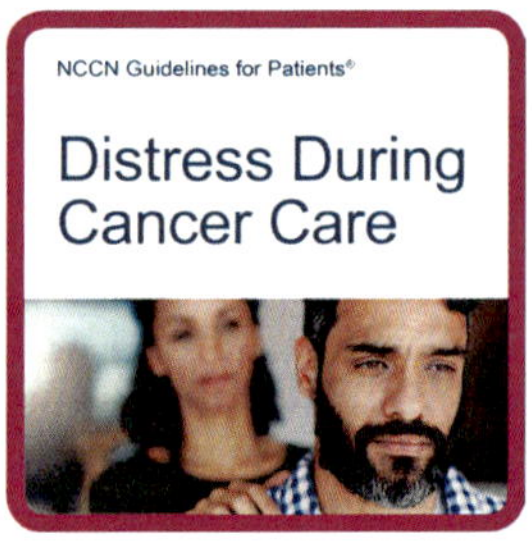

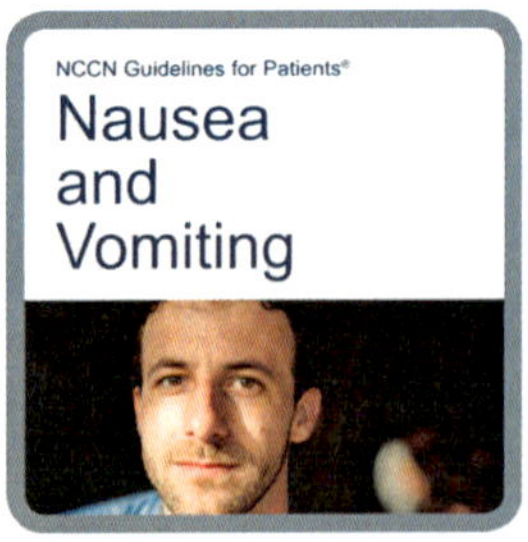

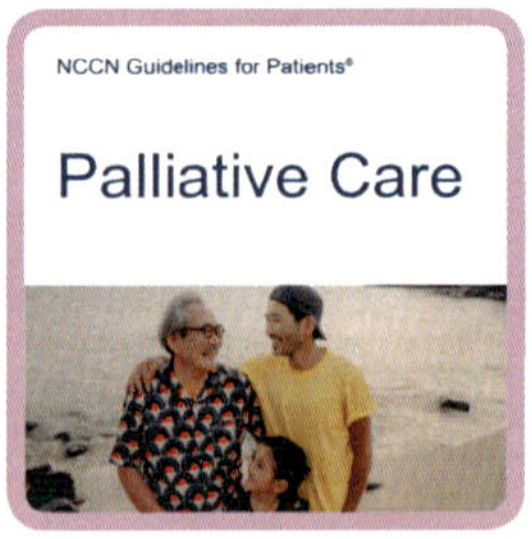

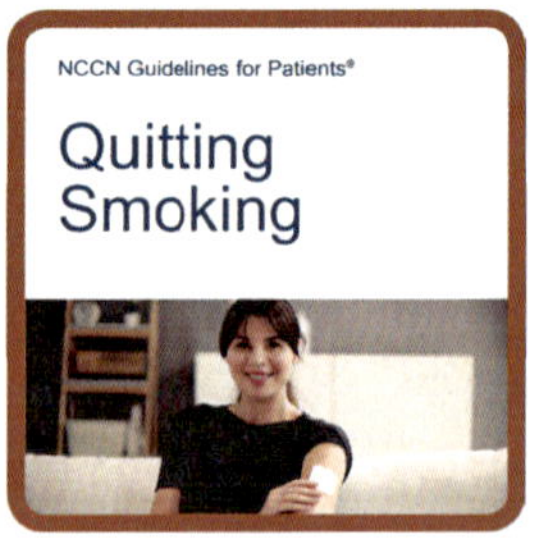

Low blood cell counts

Some cancer treatments can cause low blood cell counts.

- Anemia is a condition where the body does not have enough healthy red blood cells, resulting in less oxygen being carried to cells. Your child might feel tired easily if they are anemic.
- Neutropenia is a decrease in neutrophils, the most common type of white blood cell. These cells are important for fighting infections, and a low amount of them can increase the risk of getting an infection.
- Thrombocytopenia is a condition where there are not enough platelets in the blood. This can affect how blood clots and increase the risk of bleeding.

Managing the side effects of certain ALL treatments

This section will explain the most common side effects associated with various types of ALL drug treatments.

Steroid side effects

Sometimes steroids can cause high blood sugar, mood changes, inflammation of the pancreas (pancreatitis), or injuries to the bones. Your child's care team will monitor for these side effects and treat them. They will also check to make sure your child does not have high blood pressure (hypertension).

Vincristine side effects

Treatment with the drug vincristine can result in constipation (trouble pooping) and neuropathy (nerve problems). Neuropathy causes pain, numbness, tingling, swelling, or muscle weakness in different parts of the body. Usually, it starts in the hands or feet. Physical therapy is often used to help with these side effects.

Asparaginase chemotherapy side effects

Pegaspargase and calaspargase are a type of chemotherapy called asparaginase chemotherapy. This chemotherapy should only be given in specialized centers and hospitals. The common side effects of the chemotherapies are described below.

Hypersensitivity, allergy, and anaphylaxis
Hypersensitivity is when the immune system overreacts to a drug or substance. This can result in hives, skin welts, and trouble breathing.

An allergy is when your body reacts to a substance that is normally harmless or would not cause a response in most people. An allergic response may cause harmful symptoms, such as itching or inflammation (swelling).

Anaphylaxis or anaphylactic shock is a severe and possibly life-threatening allergic reaction.

Pancreatitis

Pancreatitis is when your pancreas becomes inflamed and swollen. This can be caused by certain medicines. If your child's pancreas becomes inflamed, treatment can be paused until the pancreas gets better.

Hemorrhage

A hemorrhage is bleeding that happens inside or outside of your body when a blood vessel is damaged. Hemorrhages can also occur in the head (this is called an intracranial hemorrhage or a brain bleed). If your child has a serious hemorrhage, treatment will be stopped until the hemorrhage is better. After that, treatment can be continued. If the hemorrhage is in their head, treatment will be stopped until the hemorrhage is gone.

Blood clots

Sometimes blood clots can break loose and travel to other parts of the body, blocking a blood vessel (called a thromboembolism). This can cause breathing problems, strokes, or other problems. If your child experiences a thromboembolism, cancer treatment will be paused, and the blood clot will be treated. Afterward, treatment can continue.

Blinatumomab and tisagenlecleucel treatment side effects

Treatments with the targeted therapy blinatumomab (Blincyto) and the CAR T-cell therapy tisagenlecleucel (Kymriah) can lead to neurologic problems (such as ICANS). Your child's care team will monitor them for these side effects, which can include confusion, tremors, drowsiness, trouble controlling muscles, seizures, or fainting.

All cancer treatments can cause unwanted health issues called side effects. It's important to tell your child's care team about all side effects so they can be managed.

Cytokine release syndrome

Cytokine release syndrome (CRS) is a condition that may occur after treatment with some types of immunotherapies, including blinatumomab and tisagenlecleucel. Signs and symptoms of CRS include fever, muscle aches, nausea, headache, rash, fast heartbeat, low blood pressure, and trouble breathing. CRS can be a serious side effect, and your child's care team will watch closely and treat your child with steroids or a drug called tocilizumab (Actemra) if they experience CRS.

> **"None of your concerns are invalid. Even if you think something is small, ask your providers. This is a way of advocating for your child."**

Helping with nutrition, emotions, pain, and more

Supportive care can also help your child with the emotions they're feeling. It can help with nutrition, pain, and other parts of care too.

Nutrition

Sometimes the symptoms of cancer or the side effects of treatment might cause your child to feel not hungry or sick to their stomach (nauseated). Healthy eating is important during treatment. It includes eating a balanced diet, eating the right amount of food, and drinking enough fluids. A registered dietitian who is an expert in nutrition and food can help. Speak to your child's care team if your child has trouble eating or if they are losing a lot of weight.

Distress

Depression, anxiety, and sleeping problems can be common among children with cancer. Talk to your child's care team about how your child might be feeling. There are services, people, and medicine that can help your child. Support and counseling services are available.

Pain

Tell your child's care team about any pain or discomfort they are feeling. Bone pain can also be common in children with ALL. Your child might meet with a pediatric pain or palliative care specialist to help manage pain.

Blood transfusions

Blood transfusions are very common during ALL treatment. A transfusion is a slow injection of blood products, such as red blood cells or platelets, into a vein.

Most blood transfusions come from blood banks. Blood is collected from strangers who donate blood. Sometimes, family members ask if they can donate blood for a family member with ALL. However, it's usually safer to use blood products from strangers than members of your own family. Your child's care team will explain more about transfusions.

Follow-up appointments

After treatment, your child's health will be monitored for side effects of treatment and the return of cancer. This is part of a care plan. It's important to keep up with any follow-up doctor visits and imaging test appointments. Find out who will coordinate your child's follow-up care.

Late side effects

Late side effects are side effects that occur months or years after a disease is diagnosed or after treatment has ended. Late effects may be caused by cancer or cancer treatment. They can include physical, mental, and social health issues and second cancers. The sooner late side effects are treated the better. Ask your child's care team about what late side effects could happen. This will help you know what to look for.

Key points

- Supportive care is health care that relieves symptoms caused by cancer or its treatment. It also helps improve quality of life.
- All cancer treatments can cause unwanted health issues called side effects. Side effects depend on many factors. These factors include the drug type and dose, length of treatment, and the person.
- Some side effects are very rare. Ask your child's care team what to expect.
- Tell your child's care team about any new or worsening symptoms they have.

Questions to ask

- What are the most common side effects of the treatments my child is going to receive? How are these side effects treated?
- What should I do if I notice changes in how my child is acting or feeling?
- What should I do if my child experiences side effects when the doctor's office isn't open?
- Will my child's care team be able to communicate with the emergency department or urgent care team?
- Who can I talk to about nutrition and what my child should be eating?

11

Other resources

Want to learn more? Here's how you can get additional help.

What else to know

This guide helps you know your child's options so you can make informed decisions and improve their cancer care. But it's not the only resource that you have.

Ask for as much information and help as you need. Many people are interested in learning more about:

- What type of ALL their child has
- The phases of ALL treatment
- Finding a doctor and cancer center that specialize in pediatric cancer
- Helping their child during treatment and care with side effects and other feelings
- Getting financial help

What else to do

Your health care center can help you with next steps. It often has on-site resources to help meet your needs and find answers to your questions. Health care centers can also inform you of resources in your community.

In addition to help from your providers, the resources listed in the next section provide support for many people like yourself.

Where to get help

Look through the list below and visit the provided websites to learn more about these organizations.

Blood & Marrow Transplant Information Network (BMT InfoNet)
bmtinfonet.org

Blood Cancer United
bloodcancerunited.org

Cancer*Care*
cancercare.org

Imerman Angels
imermanangels.org

Leukemia Research Foundation
leukemiarf.org

National Bone Marrow Transplant Link (nbmtLINK)
nbmtlink.org

NMDP
nmdp.org

Triage Cancer
triagecancer.org

Questions to ask

- Who can I talk to about help with housing, food, and other needs?
- What help is available for transportation, childcare, and home care?
- How can my child connect with others and build a support system?
- Who can I talk to if my child isn't feeling well during treatment?
- How can I reach my child's doctors after hours or on weekends?

We want your feedback!

Our goal is to provide helpful and easy-to-understand information on cancer. Take our survey to let us know what we got right and what we could do better.
NCCN.org/patients/feedback

Words to know

acute lymphoblastic leukemia (ALL)
The most common blood cancer in children. It starts in disease-fighting white blood cells called lymphocytes.

adolescent and young adult (AYA)
People who are 15 to 39 years of age at the time of initial cancer diagnosis.

***BCR::ABL1* gene**
An abnormal gene in leukemia cells formed when parts of the BCR gene and ABL1 gene join together.

bone marrow
The soft, spongy tissue in the center of most bones where blood cells are made.

bone marrow aspiration
When a small amount of liquid bone marrow is removed to test for disease.

bone marrow biopsy
When a small amount of solid bone marrow is removed to test for disease.

central nervous system
Part of the nervous system that includes the brain and spinal cord. It manages everything your child's body does.

chemotherapy
Drugs that kill fast-dividing cells, including cancer cells and normal cells.

chromosomes
Long strands of tightly packed DNA inside of cells. Chromosomes contain most of the genetic information in a cell.

clinical trial
A study of how safe and helpful tests and treatments are for people.

consolidation therapy
Often the second phase of treatment your child will get. It's given after induction therapy.

DNA
Long strands of genetic information found inside of cells.

extramedullary disease
Cancer outside of the bone marrow.

fluorescence in situ hybridization (FISH)
A lab test that uses special dyes to look for abnormal chromosomes and genes.

fusion gene
A gene made when parts of 2 separate genes join.

gene
Sections of DNA that give cells instructions for certain body functions or traits.

graft-versus-host disease (GVHD)
A disease that occurs when transplanted blood stem cells attack a person's normal cells.

hematopathologist
A doctor who uses lab tests and methods to diagnose diseases of blood cells.

hematopoietic stem cell
An immature cell in the blood and bone marrow that can develop into all types of blood cells.

hematopoietic cell transplant
A treatment that replaces damaged cells in the bone marrow with healthy, blood-forming cells. Also called a stem cell transplant or bone marrow transplant.

immune system
The body's natural defense against infection and disease.

immunotherapy
A treatment with drugs that use the immune system to fight cancer.

induction therapy
The first phase of treatment your child will receive.

infant
A child under 12 months of age.

Interfant induction therapy
The first phase of treatment for children under 12 months of age.

leukemia
A blood cancer.

lymphoblast
An immature lymphocyte (white blood cell). Also called a blast.

lymphocyte
A type of white blood cell that helps fight and prevent infections.

maintenance therapy
Usually the last phase of pediatric ALL treatment.

medullary disease
Cancer in the bone marrow.

minimal residual disease (MRD)
The small amount of cancer cells left after treatment. MRD is found by highly sensitive tests done on blood or bone marrow.

mutation
An abnormal change in a cell's DNA.

mutation testing
A test that looks for abnormal changes in genes or chromosomes.

next-generation sequencing (NGS)
A lab test used to detect abnormal changes in DNA.

pediatric
People who are 18 years of age or under at the time of a cancer diagnosis.

predisposition syndrome
An inherited genetic condition that can increase a person's chances of developing cancer.

progressive/progressing disease
The growth or spread of cancer after being tested or treated.

radiation therapy
A treatment that uses high-energy rays.

refractory cancer
When cancer doesn't get better after treatment.

regimen
A treatment plan that includes specific information about drug dose, when medicine is taken, and how long treatment will last.

relapse
When cancer comes back after it had gotten better or gone away.

remission
When the signs and symptoms of cancer have decreased or disappeared.

resistance
When cancer does not respond to a drug treatment.

steroid
A drug that can be used to reduce inflammation and kill leukemia cells.

supportive care
Treatment for the symptoms or health conditions caused by cancer or cancer treatment.

surveillance and monitoring
When your child's care team checks on them after treatment to make sure the cancer hasn't come back.

systemic therapy
Treatment that works throughout the body, such as chemotherapy.

targeted therapy
Treatment with drugs that target a specific or unique feature of cancer cells.

tyrosine kinase inhibitor (TKI)
A type of targeted therapy used to fight cancer.

share with us.

Take our survey and help make the NCCN Guidelines for Patients better for everyone!

NCCN.org/patients/comments

NCCN Contributors

This patient guide is based on the NCCN Clinical Practice Guidelines in Oncology (NCCN Guidelines®) for Pediatric Acute Lymphoblastic Leukemia, Version 1.2026. It was adapted, reviewed, and published with help from the following people:

Dorothy A. Shead, MS
Senior Director
Patient Information Operations

Megan Hollasch
Medical Writer, Patient Information

Lisa Diehl
Production Layout Artist

The NCCN Clinical Practice Guidelines in Oncology (NCCN Guidelines®) for Pediatric Acute Lymphoblastic Leukemia, Version 1.2026 were developed by the following NCCN Panel Members:

Hiroto Inaba, MD, PhD/Chair
St. Jude Children's Research Hospital/ The University of Tennessee Health Science Center

David Teachey, MD/Vice-Chair
Abramson Cancer Center at the University of Pennsylvania/ Children's Hospital of Philadelphia

Colleen Annesley, MD
Fred Hutchinson Cancer Center/ Seattle Children's Hospital

Sandeep Batra, MD
Indiana University Melvin and Bren Simon Comprehensive Cancer Center/ Riley Children's Health

Jill Beck, MD
Fred & Pamela Buffett Cancer Center/ Children's Hospital & Medical Center

*Susan Colace, MD, MSCI
The Ohio State University Comprehensive Cancer Center - James Cancer Hospital and Solove Research Institute/ Nationwide Children's Hospital

Stacy Cooper, MD
John Hopkins Kimmel Cancer Center/ Johns Hopkins Children's Center

Mari Dallas, MD
Case Comprehensive Cancer Center/ University Hospitals Seidman Cancer Center and Cleveland Clinic Taussig Cancer Institute/ University Hospitals Rainbow Babies & Children's Hospital

Satiro De Oliveira, MD
UCLA Jonsson Comprehensive Cancer Center/ UCLA Mattel Children's Hospital

Kara Kelly, MD
Roswell Park Comprehensive Cancer Center/ Roswell Park Oishei Children's Cancer and Blood Disorders Program

Carrie Kitko, MD
Vanderbilt-Ingram Cancer Center/ Monroe Carell Jr. Children's Hospital at Vanderbilt

Mira Kohorst, MD
Mayo Clinic Comprehensive Cancer Center

Matthew Kutny, MD
O'Neal Comprehensive Cancer Center at UAB/Children's of Alabama

Norman Lacayo, MD
Stanford Cancer Institute/ Lucile Packard Children's Hospital

Cathy Lee-Miller, MD
University of Wisconsin Carbone Cancer Center/ American Family Children's Hospital

Kathleen Ludwig, MD
UT Southwestern Simmons Comprehensive Cancer Center/ Children's Medical Center Dallas

Lisa Madden, MD
UC Davis Comprehensive Cancer Center

*Kelly Maloney, MD
University of Colorado Cancer Center/ Children's Hospital Colorado

David Mangum, MD
Huntsman Cancer Institute at the University of Utah/ Primary Children's Hospital

Stephanie Massaro, MD, MPH
Yale Cancer Center/Smilow Cancer Hospital/ Yale New Haven Children's Hospital

David McCall, MD
The University of Texas MD Anderson Cancer Center

*Perry Morocco, MD
The UChicago Medicine Comprehensive Cancer Center

*Brad Muller, MD
St. Jude Children's Research Hospital

Lindsey Murphy, MD, MS
City of Hope National Medical Center

Valentina Nardi, MD
Mass General Cancer Center/ Dana-Farber/Boston Children's Cancer and Blood Disorders Center

*Jenna Rossoff, MD
Robert H. Lurie Comprehensive Cancer Center of Northwestern University/Ann & Robert H. Lurie Children's Hospital of Chicago

Laura Schuettpelz, MD, PhD
Siteman Cancer Center at Barnes-Jewish Hospital and Washington University School of Medicine/ St. Louis Children's Hospital

Bijal Shah, MD
Moffitt Cancer Center

Zainab Shahid, MD, MPH
Memorial Sloan Kettering Cancer Center

Jessica Sun, MD
Duke Cancer Institute/ Duke Children's Hospital & Health Center

Victor Wong, MD
UC San Diego Moores Cancer Center/ Rady Children's Hospital-San Diego

Gregory Yanik, MD
University of Michigan Rogel Cancer Center/ C.S. Mott Children's Hospital

NCCN

Ajibola Awotiwon, MBBS, MSc
Associate Scientist/Medical Writer

Megan Lyons, MS
Oncology Scientist/Senior Medical Writer

* Reviewed this patient guide. For disclosures, visit NCCN.org/disclosures.

NCCN Cancer Centers

For contact information, visit NCCN.org/cancercenters.

Abramson Cancer Center
at the University of Pennsylvania
Philadelphia, Pennsylvania

Case Comprehensive Cancer Center/
University Hospitals Seidman Cancer Center and
Cleveland Clinic Taussig Cancer Institute
Cleveland, Ohio

City of Hope National Medical Center
Duarte, California

Dana-Farber/Brigham and Women's Cancer Center |
Mass General Cancer Center
Boston, Massachusetts

Duke Cancer Institute
Durham, North Carolina

Fox Chase Cancer Center
Philadelphia, Pennsylvania

Fred & Pamela Buffett Cancer Center
Omaha, Nebraska

Fred Hutchinson Cancer Center
Seattle, Washington

Huntsman Cancer Institute at the University of Utah
Salt Lake City, Utah

Indiana University Melvin and Bren Simon
Comprehensive Cancer Center
Indianapolis, Indiana

Johns Hopkins Kimmel Cancer Center
Baltimore, Maryland

Mayo Clinic Comprehensive Cancer Center
Phoenix/Scottsdale, Arizona
Jacksonville, Florida
Rochester, Minnesota

Memorial Sloan Kettering Cancer Center
New York, New York

Moffitt Cancer Center
Tampa, Florida

O'Neal Comprehensive Cancer Center at UAB
Birmingham, Alabama

Robert H. Lurie Comprehensive Cancer Center
of Northwestern University
Chicago, Illinois

Roswell Park Comprehensive Cancer Center
Buffalo, New York

Siteman Cancer Center at Barnes-Jewish Hospital
and Washington University School of Medicine
St. Louis, Missouri

St. Jude Children's Research Hospital/
The University of Tennessee Health Science Center
Memphis, Tennessee

Stanford Cancer Institute
Stanford, California

The Ohio State University Comprehensive Cancer Center -
James Cancer Hospital and Solove Research Institute
Columbus, Ohio

The UChicago Medicine Comprehensive Cancer Center
Chicago, Illinois

The University of Texas MD Anderson Cancer Center
Houston, Texas

UC Davis Comprehensive Cancer Center
Sacramento, California

UC San Diego Moores Cancer Center
La Jolla, California

UCLA Jonsson Comprehensive Cancer Center
Los Angeles, California

UCSF Helen Diller Family Comprehensive Cancer Center
San Francisco, California

University of Colorado Cancer Center
Aurora, Colorado

University of Michigan Rogel Cancer Center
Ann Arbor, Michigan

University of Wisconsin Carbone Cancer Center
Madison, Wisconsin

UT Southwestern Simmons
Comprehensive Cancer Center
Dallas, Texas

Vanderbilt-Ingram Cancer Center
Nashville, Tennessee

Yale Cancer Center/Smilow Cancer Hospital
New Haven, Connecticut

Index

Made in United States
North Haven, CT
17 October 2026

20523722R00046